The Thirteen Months of Pregnancy

A Guide for the Pregnant Father

The Thirteen Months of Pregnancy

A Guide for the Pregnant Father

By

BILL M. ATALLA

with

Steve Beitler

Illustrated by

Marduk Sayad

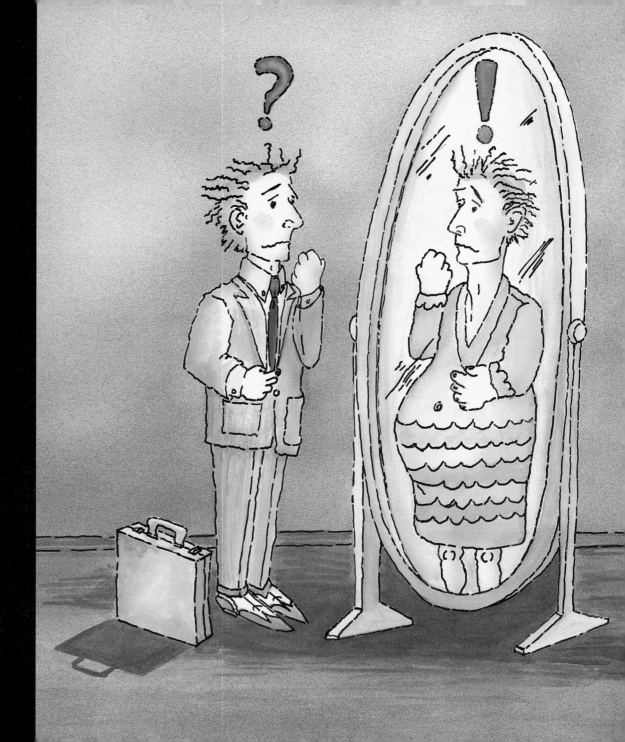

The Thirteen Months of **Pregnancy** *A Guide for the Pregnant Father*
By **Bill M. Atalla**
with Steve Beitler

Published by
o]**aly**
EnOuGh
P.O. Box 1213
Kenwood, California 95452

Copyright © 1992 Bill M. Atalla

Publisher's Cataloging-in-Publication Data

Atalla, Bill M.

The Thirteen Months of Pregnancy: *A Guide for the Pregnant Father* / Bill M. Atalla with Steve Beitler

p cm.

Includes bibliographical references (p.) and glossary.

1. Pregnancy—Male experience. 2. Fatherhood—Prenatal, labor, delivery, postpartum, early months after delivery.

3. Parenting—Male experience during the early months after delivery. 4. Relationships—Male experience with mother and child during pregnancy and early months after delivery. 5. Childbirth—Male experience. I. Beitler, Steve D., 1948-. II. Title.

618.2 - dc20 92-060038

ISBN 0-9631754-5-9: $19.95 Hardcover

Printed in Mexico

10 9 8 7 6 5 4 3 2 1

DEDICATION

This book is dedicated to my wife Carolyn,
who is always my inspiration.
To my daughters, Tiffany and Ashley,
who allow me the opportunity
to be a child again and encourage me to be a great father.

ACKNOWLEDGMENTS

A special thank you to those listed who contributed directly to the quality of this book. Your insights and support were invaluable. Thank you is also in order to the many fathers and expectant mothers and fathers who have validated this work for those yet to follow.

Kathleen Archambeau, Dr. Martin Atalla, Dorothy Berry, Pamela D'Angelo, Trevor Glenn II, Gina Renée Gross, Lauretta Habermeyer, Dr. Steve Heidorn, David Lowe, and Dr. Paul Madsen.

CONTENTS

PREFACE

This book is the only one you'll ever read on pregnancy that you'll want to read again. It's written for men, by men, in a way that's easy to understand and contains plenty of mission-critical information.

Most books about pregnancy treat men as innocent bystanders whose "job is done." My book puts men at center stage. That's because the difference between how you and your wife experience pregnancy is more than just physical—it's emotional, too.

You may be wondering if I've miscalculated how long pregnancy lasts. I haven't. It still takes about nine months from conception to birth . . . but I also believe that the real adjustment to being a father happens after another four months. A thirteen-month pregnancy takes you and your wife beyond carrying time to caring time.

My goal is to help you not only endure, but enjoy, pregnancy. I'll show you ways you can help your wife—and yourself—that go far beyond yelling "Push!" when the big moment arrives. If you're a decisive and proactive man to whom participation makes more sense than sliding through on instinct and hoping for the best, then this book is for you. It's designed for men who want to work with their wives as equal partners on the road to parenthood.

If you're looking for the straight scoop from a book that won't waste your time, you've found it. If you're a nineties man looking for balance among family, work, and your personal life, but aren't sure how to achieve it, I've got some ideas for you.

I'll also describe how a couple's relationship changes and grows throughout pregnancy, resulting in a new and multidimensional family relationship.

As you've watched that stack of books on your wife's nightstand grow, you've both probably known all along that you'll never read them. Relax. *The Thirteen Months of Pregnancy* is the only book you need to read. It gives men the play by play without the extraneous details.

The book advances chronologically through the pregnancy, and highlights five phases you are most likely to experience. These phases brief you on what you need to know and when, in order to enjoy this new experience. For as you're about to discover, *thirteen* is anything but unlucky.

Introduction

Launching a Family

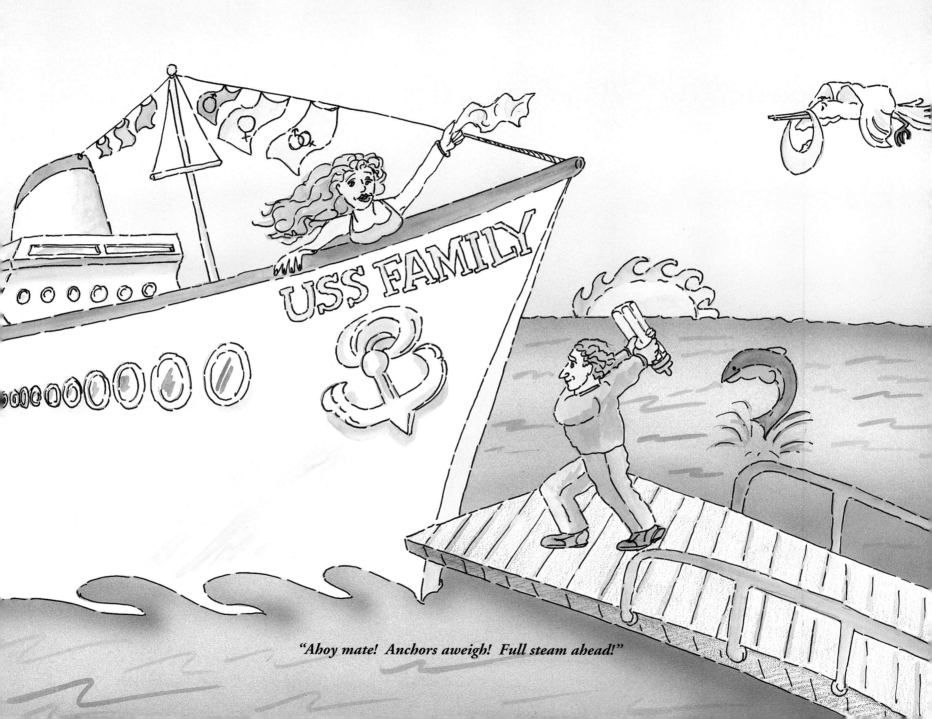

"Ahoy mate! Anchors aweigh! Full steam ahead!"

"Face it—you're as pregnant as your wife." My friend's words hit me like a sucker punch. But where a right hand from nowhere would have knocked my lights out, that comment switched one on.

I'd known for about six weeks that I was going to be a father—long enough to get over the first jolt but not long enough to feel comfortable. I felt distant from my wife, who was getting all the attention. I was happy about becoming a father, but worried, too.

My friend's remark motivated me to start making pregnancy what I wanted it to be—something positive, maybe even fun—not scary.

The Thirteen Months of Pregnancy is for any man who feels isolated, overwhelmed, or even frightened by the reality of becoming a father. This book cuts through tons of information, advice, and folklore on pregnancy to hone in on what you need in a way that respects your time and intelligence. After all, time is money—and you're going to need all you can get of both in the next thirteen months.

I cover sex, work, the transition to family life, and sex some more. I talk about the physical and emotional roller-coaster your wife is on and include status updates on your baby-to-be. I present the entire experience of pregnancy from a man's perspective, and show you how to reap the benefits of being actively involved during these thirteen months.

I also suggest ways for you not only to take (some) control over what's happening in your life but to make pregnancy enjoyable for you and your wife. You have a better chance at enjoying pregnancy than your wife because you're not carrying the child; and I promise, she'll remind you of this many times over the next few months. But you can minimize her discomfort through understanding—and active participation.

I have two daughters, ages seven and ten. In the eighties, I made a rapid climb up the corporate ladder, becoming CEO of a Silicon Valley electronics firm that I eventually sold to a larger Fortune 500 computer company. By then I'd had all I wanted of the executive suite, and I left the company to devote more attention to my young family.

I didn't know it at the time, but I had become a pioneer in the trend of the nineties. Today more men are reexamining what success really means, and they're redefining it in terms of the quality of their family lives. Money isn't the only measure of success any more.

If you think pregnancy means worry, physical discomfort for your wife, and marital tension, you're right. But it's much more, and I can help you discover the positive and rewarding aspects.

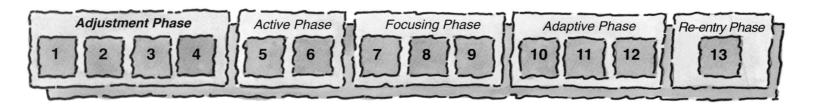

The "Adjustment" Phase

Welcome to your new life, Dad! During the first four months of pregnancy (chapters I-IV), the smartest thing to do is let the news settle in and work closely with your wife.

She's adjusting both physically and emotionally; your adjustment is probably just emotional. But you shouldn't assume that makes it any easier. You're likely to feel bombarded by memories, feelings, and thoughts that enter your mind without any apparent explanation. But there is an explanation—you're going to be a father!

This section describes common reactions men have to getting the big news. It provides updates on the physical symptoms your wife may experience. It gives you guidance on some key early decisions, such as what sort of childbirth you want and how to get ready at home and work. You might feel a little overwhelmed in these early months, so it's important to be patient with yourself and your wife from the beginning.

Every minute of pregnancy isn't a peak experience. But the right blend of attitude, knowledge, and effort can:

- **strengthen the ties between you and your wife**
- **create a solid foundation for your new family**
- **prepare you for parenthood**
- **help you achieve balance among family, career, and personal life.**

This book will show you how to realize these benefits. Because you're as pregnant as your wife. But you don't have to face it alone. There are lots of successful fathers out there, and my goal is to help you join their fraternity.

Chapter One

The Big News

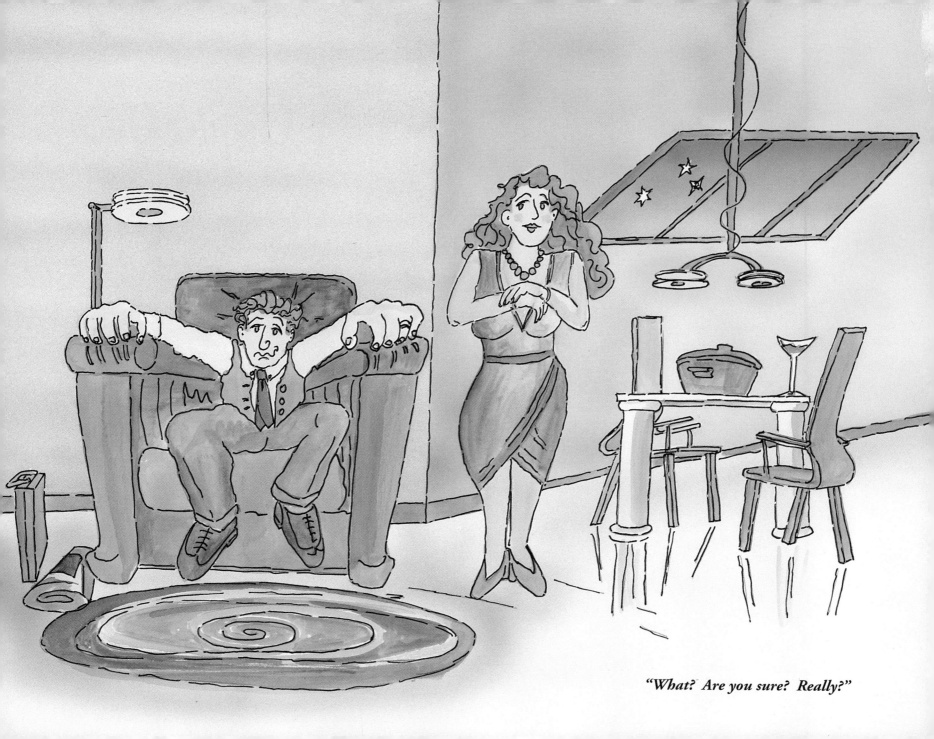

"What? Are you sure? Really?"

For all your wonderful qualities, Dad, you're probably not a medical trailblazer. It's still your wife who's physically pregnant. (Be thankful for that!)

But as a father-to-be you're a good bet to have feelings—and maybe even physical changes—that are as intense as your wife's. Some of these feelings are similar to hers; others are yours alone.

There's a scene from "I Love Lucy" that illustrates this well. Ricky is leading his Cuban All-Stars on the bandstand. Between numbers the headwaiter passes him a note. It's a request for a song to help someone in the crowd celebrate some great news—a woman is having a baby.

It's soon clear who's pregnant—Lucy! But it takes Ricky a while to catch on. Then he looks more surprised than if he'd met an alien. He's dazed. He's confused. *He's pregnant.*

How Do You React?

Even if your pregnancy is planned, the news of your new arrival probably caught you off guard.

Ambivalence is a common reaction. You're happy, proud, and feel a surge of closeness to your wife. But there's some apprehension, too.

Can you afford it? Is it really the right time? Will your wife lose her figure? Will you be a good father? What about the economy, your career, your travel plans? Will spontaneity be just a memory for you and your wife?

Don't worry! (That's always good advice for fathers-to-

be.) Those concerns and feelings are completely normal.

Researchers have taken a close look at first reactions to finding out there's a baby coming. Women are often enthusiastic, as well as concerned about how their husbands will react. "What happens if he doesn't really want a child?" Many women are reassured by knowing that their friends, sisters, and mothers are eager to help. Newly pregnant women often get more self-involved. They're fascinated by the life growing within them and pay closer attention to their bodies and moods. And unlike men, women often have their support network already in place—relatives and friends who have children and are happy to share their experiences.

So right out of the gate, you're coping with your own questions and dealing with new behavior in your wife. Whether you are shocked, overjoyed, confused, overwhelmed, or feeling a combination of a few feelings, don't fight those feelings. Realize that you are reacting to a new situation in your life, one that you may not have expected. Your feelings aren't unique, and many men feel stress, fear, and ecstasy when they imagine the pitter-patter of little feet . . . just like you.

What should you do? For starters, talk about your feelings! Let your wife know what's on your mind; encourage her to do the same. Don't let a small worry get out of control by keeping it bottled up. But plenty of men do just that. One study identified seven fears about pregnancy and fatherhood that men are likely to keep to themselves. Do any of these ring true with you?

1) **The birth process; will you be able to keep it together during labor and delivery?**
2) **Money.**
3) **Obstetrics and gynecology; will you really have to go to the doctor with your wife?**
4) **Paternity; almost half your counterparts in the study expressed concern over whether they were really the father.**
5) **Fear of losing your wife or child, their health, or well-being.**
6) **Worries about your relationship with your wife; when you're parents, will you ever be a couple again?**
7) **Greater awareness of your own mortality.**

The key to handling these issues, and others, is to get past any embarrassment you feel. Talk to your wife, your friends, your brothers and sisters and parents. It turned out I had lots of male friends who were not only willing, but eager, to talk about their pregnancies and early fatherhood. It's reassuring to hear people you respect tell you that they had concerns similar to what you may now be feeling. Who knows? You may even start an expectant male support group!

Your Due Date

There are two formulas for calculating your expected date of delivery, or as it is commonly referred to, "due date." First:
- Determine the first day of your wife's last menstrual period.
- Add seven days.
- Subtract three months.

Or perhaps you'd prefer this simpler method:
- Add five months to the time you first feel your baby move.

Keep in mind that these formulas are only estimates and it is not uncommon for a baby to be born two weeks before or after this date.

I recall, we held this date in high regard, and as it neared, everything we did was centered around it. However my first child was two weeks late and the second one was four weeks early. As you can see, these formulas are clearly approximations.

On the Physical Front

Your wife is also likely to have some physical reactions that could surprise you.

First is the classic morning sickness—I learned plenty about this first-hand. The stereotype is that women experience nonstop nausea and vomiting every morning for the first two to three months they're pregnant.

The reality is often different. Only 30-50 percent of pregnant women ever experience morning sickness. And the term is misleading, since newly pregnant women can get sick anytime.

It's not clear what causes morning sickness, although some people believe emotional factors play a role. You needn't worry about morning sickness hurting the baby unless it's so bad that it interferes with normal nutrition. And it's unusual for morning sickness to persist beyond the third month, though there are exceptions.

Can you help your wife prevent or cure morning sickness? Probably not. But there are steps your wife can take to improve the odds:

- **Eat a high-protein, high-carbohydrate diet—both help fight nausea.**
- **Drink a lot of fluids.**
- **Avoid sights and smells that produce queasiness.**
- **Eat before feeling hungry.**
- **Don't bounce out of bed the second after waking up.**
- **Check with your doctor about vitamins or other supplements that can help.**

At the other extreme, it's sometimes not just the woman who displays "symptoms" in early pregnancy. There's a small number of men who start to feel queasy in the morning if their wives are battling morning sickness. They might get headaches or lose their appetite. When men display these "sympathetic symptoms" of pregnancy it's called *couvade*. It's not clear what causes couvade, but a surprising number of men experience it, and you shouldn't panic if this starts happening to you. Relax and remember that it's only temporary. In most cases—like morning sickness itself—time is the cure.

Sick . . . and Tired?

Even if your wife avoids morning sickness, it's likely that she'll feel tired often. Why? A pregnant body is like a factory at full capacity, and that's a strain. So try to help your wife get to bed earlier at night. Let her stay in bed longer. Maybe even encourage her to take it easy and nap during the day. If that means you get your own breakfast, run a few extra errands, or make dinner a few times a week, do it.

The Longer View

Before we get further into the details of what to look for and do in the early months of pregnancy, let's step back for a minute.

Pregnancy is more than a collection of new tasks and experiences. It's a whole new life—for you, your wife, and your relationship. It's a change that will demand adjustment, negotiation, tolerance, and patience. And sometimes that extra large dose of TLC.

A change like this also calls for a *strategy*. Having been

through it twice, and having learned the hard way, I'd suggest you consider these four points in devising yours:

1) Parents-to-be are going through a "rite of passage" from which they emerge with a new identity.

You've never been a parent before. You'll never be childless again. That's a change you shouldn't underestimate.

Many fathers-to-be see the upcoming birth as the close of a chapter in their lives. Just as getting married may have put an end to four nights a week of "hanging out with the guys" or playing in three basketball leagues every season.

That might be a major shift for you. Those sixty to seventy-hour work weeks and hectic travel schedules can start to make less sense. But you can't abandon your career. And you still need time for yourself and for you and your wife as a couple.

Welcome to the basic dilemma of being a father in the nineties! The good news is that plenty of men, myself included, have faced this challenge and conquered it. You will, too. It takes time, but can you name anything truly worthwhile that happens overnight?

Take a minute to examine your attitude. Is it as positive and supportive as it could be? It's just as easy to see pregnancy as the beginning of an exciting adventure rather than the end of one.

2) Active involvement in pregnancy can strengthen your relationship, make you a better parent, and calm your nerves.

Pregnancy is like many things you do: Investing time and energy brings rewards. Involvement helps your wife have an easier pregnancy and prepares you both to be parents when the baby arrives.

And there's another payoff. Parents-to-be who tackle pregnancy together add depth to their bond that nothing else can match. In the short term, this means a faster return to the "romantic" part of your relationship after your baby is born. And over the long haul, your active involvement will pay dividends when your child leaves home and it's just you and your wife again. (That's what I call the "long-term bond" market in pregnancy.)

3) Knowledge is power.

Knowledge is the best antidote to fear and doubt. The more you know about pregnancy, the more confidence you'll develop. But I'm not suggesting you bury yourself in the library—who has the time? Some carefully selected reading (starting with this book) and talking with your wife's doctor are a good way to start. (We'll look more closely at your relationship with your wife's medical team in chapter III.)

Knowing what lies ahead for you and your wife allows you to make realistic plans. Knowledge gives you the power to adapt to the upcoming changes. It allows you both to make the necessary adjustments in your everyday life, as the pregnancy experience unfolds.

4) Teamwork is everything; there's no "I" in "parent."

Experienced parents know that raising children requires consistent teamwork that makes a high-wire act look sloppy. Do you compete with or complement your wife when it comes to work around the house or in the garden?

Parenting requires both a new level and a new kind of teamwork with your wife. Something you may not be used to experiencing. Be ready to upgrade your dish washing, cooking, and housecleaning skills. Get comfortable improvising and staying flexible. Be ready to display the patience of a Mother Teresa. Only then will you have what it takes to be a great parenting partner with your wife. I'm not suggesting that you put on an apron

and abandon your former life; pitching in with whatever needs to be done goes a long way. Your caring and help will allow your wife to face the day more positively.

The bottom line? Thoreau never had children, but he might have been talking about pregnancy when he said, "This time, like all other times, is a very good one if we but know what to do with it."

Relationship Update

Assessing your relationship with your wife can help you and your spouse remain close during pregnancy. It is a way to avoid or resolve misunderstandings that can arise if either of you keep your feelings bottled up. I'll use illustrations throughout this book to help you visualize what you may experience in your relationship.

Pregnancy is a paradox. It's one of the most joyous yet stressful events any couple can experience. It can tax even the strongest relationship and is rarely the way to make a faulty one better. Even the best relationships are temporarily stressed during your thirteen-month journey through pregnancy.

Your active involvement in this traditionally "female" event can add depth and strength to the bond with your spouse. The efforts you both make to communicate, to stay focused on common goals, and to respect each other's individuality will pay dividends during these months and for years to come.

The goals and values you have as individuals should already overlap in a number of areas and the baby should not become the only area of commonalty.

Action

Remember the two of you are a team and that communication is vital to maintain your couple's relationship. Agreement as to your goals, values, and priorities is important. Be prepared that pregnancy might change some of them. Discuss your thoughts and feelings regarding these changes, openly and often.

Chapter Two

Foreign Territory

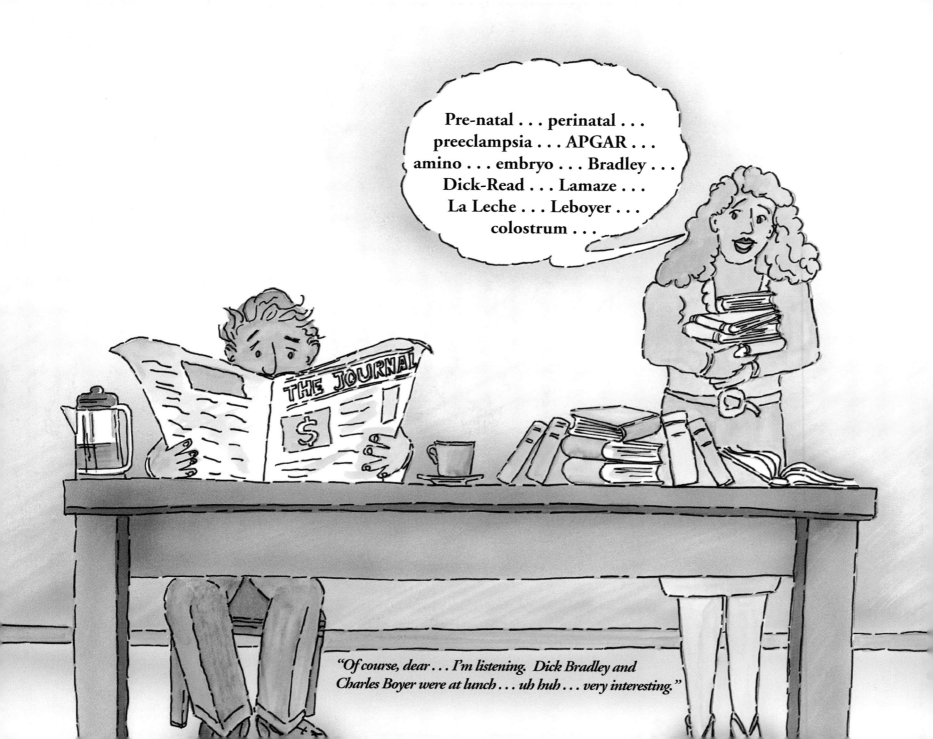

Pregnancy changes your whole focus on life. And I thank my daughters every day for those changes.

But when you first learn you're going to be a father, it *can* be overwhelming.

This chapter describes issues—and opportunities—you might encounter in the aftermath of the big news. It looks at two big pieces of your life: your career and spousal relationship.

Money and Work

On average, about 4.32 seconds elapse between your finding out that you're having a baby and you or your wife asking, "Can we afford it?"

For couples who haven't been salting away a fortune or haven't won the lottery, looking at higher expenses—and maybe a lower income (if your wife is working)—can be frightening.

So . . . should your wife be the one to put her career on hold? If so, how long will she stay home with the baby? Will she want to go back to work? When?

Those are big issues. I found myself worrying about pregnancy causing a nasty "chain reaction." As a commissioned sales executive, I was spending a tremendous amount of time on the road, keeping my current clients happy and finding new ones. My income was directly related to that travel, and less time on the road would mean less money. I was able to make some adjustments to prevent a steep drop in income, and you can do the same thing—here's how.

Financial Fundamentals

A newborn may not know anything about finances, but your child will teach you more about economics than any professor.

When you're a parent, expenses fall into two categories: those you anticipate and those you don't. Some men figure the answer is simple—more money. They take on a second job or start to look for a better one.

More money helps, but a new child puts your time and energy at a premium. A second job could strain you to the breaking point. If your goal is to balance career, family, and personal life, a second job doesn't make sense.

Let's put one big myth to rest right here. The eighties notion of quality time misses the point. I advocate *quantity* time. Why? Because the real fun of being a parent, and the lasting bond between parent and child, can only be experienced and forged over time—lots of time. I think I understood this instinctively when I decided to drop out of the rat race (which can't be won) and spend more time with my family.

Research supports this notion as well. A Harvard study of children ranging from newborns to eighteen months old showed that quantity, not "quality," is what counts when it comes to spending time with your child.

It's easy to show up for recitals and graduations. It's harder—but more rewarding—to put in the less exciting hours. But that's when the real work of parenting gets done.

And it's amazing—even the most routine task takes on new meaning when your baby is part of it.

Beyond Time and Money

A sensible approach to getting beyond the time-and-money dilemma starts with financial planning and a career assessment.

The steps are simple. You need to look at how much money is coming in and how much is going out . . . and a very close look at where it's going. The word is budget.

A little more attention to your spending returns big dividends. The trick is focused spending, in effect, you and your wife asking yourselves repeatedly, "Do we really need it or do we just want it?" Does it really make sense to buy that sports car you've always wanted, or would a station wagon or minivan be smarter?

Here's another trick: Don't make any major purchase without "sleeping on it." Give yourselves twenty-four hours after you decide to spring for something to let your decision settle in. It might look different in the morning.

The start of pregnancy is the best time to work on new ways of looking at your finances and spending. Being a parent forces choices on you only if you don't make them yourself.

The good thing is that you're going to be much more willing to make those choices when you see your beautiful new baby. It didn't seem possible to me either, but I'll promise you that's when you'll be eager to start saving for college and shopping for your child's clothes, toys, and more.

Career Assessment

Is your career on track? Are you successful at work? Do you enjoy what you do?

Beyond that paycheck, are you getting the other rewards —a sense of accomplishment, recognition, personal and professional growth—that are so important?

Pregnant or not, these are important issues. But let's get something straight. Pregnancy isn't the right time for a new job. You should wait at least until the baby is born.

This is as close as I come to an iron law of pregnancy. Actually, this is just part of the larger (and, I promise, the only) strict rule of pregnancy. This rule states: "No big changes on any major fronts of your life—no job shifts, no house-buying, no career changes."

I learned this the hard way. I felt energized by our big news. I felt really positive about the change and decided that this would be a good time to expand my business and my responsibilities by establishing new sales offices around the world. Unfortunately, it worked. Expansion quickly put me on a steep learning curve and a heavy travel program. Eighty-hour weeks became the norm.

The result? The business grew fast, but I didn't have the time or energy to participate in many important events in my wife's pregnancy. When I wasn't there I wound up disappointing both of us, as well as adding to my confusion, guilt, and anger. (Part of my reason for writing this book is to help other men avoid this mistake.)

Why are you working so hard in the first place? For your family! And your family starts when you know you're going to have a baby—not when the baby arrives.

If pregnancy is a good time to do a nuts-and-bolts inventory of your finances, it's also a great time to step back and assess your career and where you're headed. Just don't act right now if your career assessment reveals that it's time to move on. Put the drastic changes on hold—don't turn up the stress by piling a new job on top of pregnancy.

Your Wife's Career Is Also Important!

What will your role be in caring for your newborn? You don't have to map out a plan within hours of finding out that you're going to be a parent. But you don't want to first raise the topic as you're driving home from the hospital either.

If your wife doesn't work, and your last name isn't Rockefeller, she's the logical choice for staying home after your baby arrives. But you're not off the hook, Dad. No matter who works or who stays home, parenting means significant adjustments for both of you.

What I said about your career assessment applies to your wife if she's working. Start by taking a good look, together, at both your careers. Don't assume your wife will be the one who puts hers on hold. Even if that's the way to go, take some time to find out how she feels. Should she take three months off? More? Less? Is going back part-time a possibility? A reality?

Don't you feel better when you've had a hand in a decision that affects you? The same applies to pregnancy. The time you spend in mutual decision-making, even for the easier calls (there aren't many), will help you and your wife build a new level of closeness with each other.

Just Between You and Your Wife

Some men feel distant from their newly pregnant wives just when their wives feel closer to their husbands.

Wives go through physical changes and the same apprehensions as their husbands over money, their fitness to be parents, labor, and childbirth. They've never had a greater need for the emotional support that only you can provide.

Coping with this irony is a major priority for the first weeks, or months, of pregnancy. Be active! Talk to each other, to friends, to doctors, to people at work, to parents, and to brothers, sisters, or in-laws.

The distance that stress creates can easily be bridged with a little extra sparkle and romance. How about "dating" your wife again? Try coming home a bit early from work and preparing a candlelight dinner for two. Bring her flowers. Treat her to a bubble bath and sensuous massage . . . Who knows? You may even get one in return. No matter how seemingly little the acts you take seem to you, remember that they can have an extra special effect on your relationship at this time in your pregnancy.

And don't forget communication in your intimacy. Try spending a quiet night alone simply *talking,* confiding in one another about your goals and dreams . . . or perhaps some of the frustrations and obstacles that you never dreamed you'd encounter during this period. If you're not ready for soul-searching at the end of a long day, remember that idle conversation never hurt anyone . . . especially while sitting on the patio gazing at the stars.

What Else Can You Do?

• Take time for things that are meaningful to both of you. Have dinner at that restaurant you've wanted to get back to, stroll on the beach, go to a movie—anything that's rewarding and romantic for both of you. It's a great way to build togetherness in these early months.

• Spend time with friends who are new parents. (You don't have to be there when they get home from the hospital.) After their initial adjustment period, many new parents crave some connection with their former lifestyles. You may be shocked at what you see—your old sports-fanatic friend raving about his new baby with the enthusiasm he used to have for that last-second winning shot from center court. Your friend's new behavior may seem strange, but that could be you in just nine months.

• Start a self-improvement program together. If you've wanted to break an old habit, improve your diet, or exercise regularly, there's no better incentive than becoming parents. As always, check with your doctor first on any new exercise or nutrition program. And start slowly. You might want to dust off your tennis rackets or join one of those health clubs that's always offering a discount for new members. You'll improve your health while you're getting into good habits for your child to model.

There is another activity that can provide emotional and physical closeness. . . .

Sex and the Newly Pregnant

Being pregnant intensifies the emotional needs of both newly expecting parents. Sex would seem to be the perfect way to meet those needs. But you might not be in the mood! (I can almost hear you saying, "I doubt it.")

Your wife may be tired. She may be nauseous. She's probably urinating frequently. Her breasts are swollen and tender, and her moods can swing pretty wildly and often. (Isn't this a scary picture?)

Not a sure bet to inflame your passion. What's more, you might be grappling with ambivalence and apprehension about becoming a father, which could dampen your desire for intimacy even more.

The result? The "typical" pattern is for sexual activity to decrease during the first three months, pick up during the middle three months, and then fall off again in the final three months. In the early weeks of pregnancy, this might suit you fine, since you're still getting used to the changing shape of your wife (and life). You might also have some fears about causing a miscarriage, inducing labor, or harming the baby.

In fact, under practically all circumstances, intercourse won't hurt the baby. It can't infect or crush the baby because the developing baby is protected by a bag of fluid called the amniotic sac. By this time the baby is firmly anchored to the uterus, so intercourse shouldn't cause a miscarriage.

But there are circumstances under which sexual activity is out of the question. If your wife has any bleeding, you should refrain from sex and check with your doctor immediately. If your wife has had a miscarriage, ask your doctor, who may suggest abstaining for a few months, when the pregnancy is more firmly established.

But if your wife isn't experiencing any of these limiting conditions, intercourse during pregnancy can be pleasurable. It could even give both of you the emotional support and sheer physical enjoyment that words can't convey. And who knows? You could be one of the lucky couples for whom pregnancy makes having sex more exciting. Maybe it's the freedom from birth control. Or the novelty. Who's to question?

The Bottom Line

When it comes to sex and the newly pregnant, you need patience, sensitivity, and flexibility. These qualities are virtues throughout your thirteen-month journey. When they're combined with knowledge, teamwork, and a positive, energetic approach, there are very few obstacles pregnancy can put in your path. Work and your relationship are important all the time, but especially during pregnancy. Your concerns about them are likely to escalate as the months roll on, so I'll continue to focus on them.

Thoughts for the Early Months

• Observe your spending more closely. You might want to keep a spending diary; for now, get in the habit of keeping closer tabs on where your money goes.

• If you don't already consult a financial planner or accountant, start to recruit one; word of mouth is the best way. Professional help in putting together your financial strategy can help you clarify your goals and what it will take to achieve them.

• Take stock of your career. Look ahead at what will be required of you over the next year. What priorities will allow you to make the most of your time at work? Pregnancy and fatherhood put many new demands on your limited time.

• Think of and follow through on ways to reaffirm your relationship with your wife. Share your feelings and concerns and encourage her to do the same. Focusing on your relationship with your wife during pregnancy is a key to becoming a great parenting team—and communication between the two of you is vital.

Your Baby's First Two Months

The baby is approximately one inch long and weighs about two grams by the end of the second month of pregnancy. Even at this size, your baby is starting to emerge.

The developing brain and head are disproportionately large, and the reproductive organs are visible, but not so well formed as to be able to tell the sex. What had been an embryo is rapidly becoming a fetus (your baby).

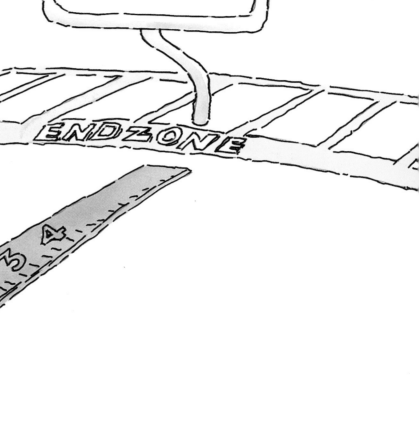

Relationship Update

It is quite common during pregnancy for the man to feel removed and distant from his wife's attention and affection. This distance can become an issue for men during the middle months. Your wife is focusing on the baby, her changing body, and her capabilities about becoming a mother. She's often the center of positive attention with friends and family who want to talk about . . . the baby. While on the other hand you are receiving comments from fathers that are sometimes less than encouraging.

To top things off she's probably not feeling sexy or particularly attractive. How could you not feel distant?

If you feel this distance, take the initiative to reaffirm your involvement in the pregnancy. Typically this situation is temporary. Knowing this, it is your goal to minimize the distance during this time. Often discussion alone can cause mutual awareness which is the beginning of bringing you back into this developing family picture.

Action

Take time to remove your wife from the day to day environment. Arrange a relaxing atmosphere to discuss your feelings and needs as well as hers. Do these with the goal in mind to remain a close and supportive partner during this pregnancy. Discussion beyond your baby with emphasis on your goals as a couple is significant and beneficial. They will result in pulling each of you closer together. Also reassure your wife how sexy and appealing she is and how much you appreciate her "new beauty."

Chapter Three

Decisions, Decisions

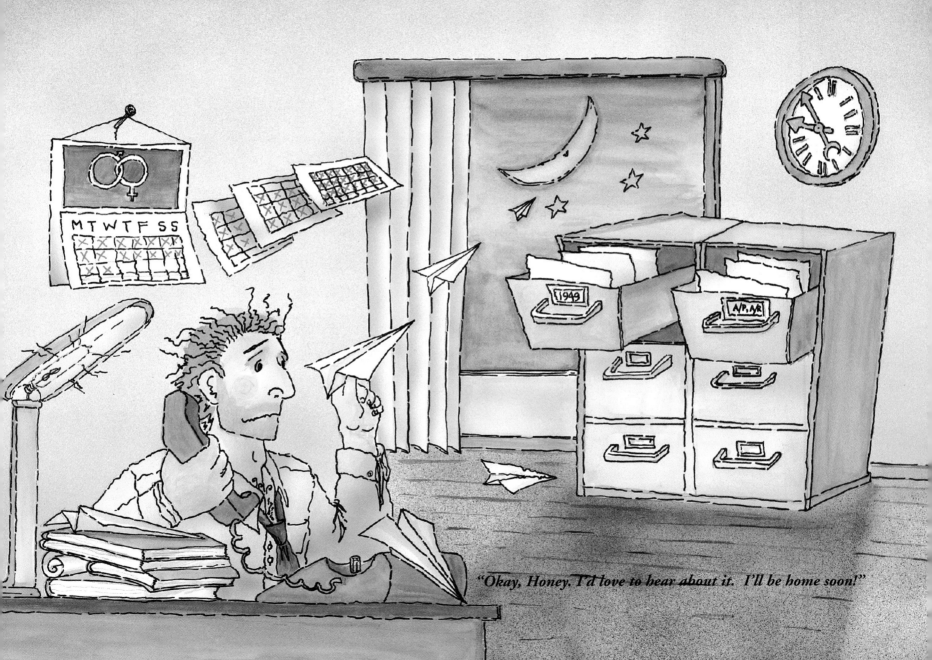

"Okay, Honey. I'd love to hear about it. I'll be home soon!"

Although you are changing, feeling, and experiencing some rather weighty decisions right now, try to lighten up and have some fun with this once-in-a-lifetime experience. Now is your opportunity to be creative and inventive in sharing the news. You need only to decide how and when.

I know people who have sent their out-of-town friends telegrams. My wife and I have friends who composed wacky messages, complete with background music and appropriate baby sounds, to leave on phone machines.

You can have fun sharing the news in different ways. It makes sense to tailor your approach to your audience. You may want to put together a list of close friends and business associates, but be sure to contact your family first! Don't forget to tell those grandparents-to-be personally, and early, since it's their sacred mission in life to spoil your child mercilessly.

But not too early. Why not give yourself and your wife a little time to let the news settle in? Pregnancy is a thirteen-month transition to a new you. You both deserve time to adjust. Savoring your secret for a little while is harmless fun and can produce a surge of closeness between you and your wife. In addition, you probably don't want the news to travel too far, too fast, just in case something endangers or ends the pregnancy. You may feel more

secure by letting your pregnancy get firmly established before you tell the whole world.

But you can't wait too long. Your wife, after all, will want to wear maternity clothes before people start wondering if she's getting fat. She may even enjoy this way of proudly showing the world she's pregnant.

The Right Person for the Job

If you owned a $175,000 sports car, would you let the kid down the street fix it?

The same applies to pregnancy. You wouldn't let the checkout clerk at the supermarket or even your mother-in-law tell you how to run your business. Although that may not stop either of them from offering plenty of advice. And you're not going to pick your doctor out of the phone book.

Choosing your main medical practitioner—obstetrician, midwife, or family practitioner—is part of a larger decision: What type of childbirth do you want? You and your wife have many of options. These range from the "standard" hospital birth, with a dazzling array of fetal monitors, intravenous rigs, and other high-tech equipment on hand, to having your baby at home the "natural" way. And there are other choices that combine elements of both.

In this chapter, I'll try to help you and your wife through decisions on the "who" (will deliver your child) and the "where" (hospital, birth center, home) of the event that will launch you into fatherhood.

It's a little like planning your wedding—the earlier you make these choices the better. It takes time to develop good rapport with your medical team. It takes time to work out the details about delivery. And it takes time for your practitioner to know you and your wife, especially her medical history and feelings about what she wants childbirth to be like. As with practically everything in pregnancy, these decisions aren't as simple as "this is right and that's wrong." What's right is what makes you and your wife comfortable and confident.

And remember, no matter what kind of birth you choose, the late twentieth century is the best time in all history (from the standpoint of health and safety) to have a baby. If you do your homework, help your partner stay healthy and fit, and approach childbirth with confidence, the odds are strongly in your favor that your pregnancy experience will be a rewarding one.

First Things First

Before planning for birth, there's one thing to do. Check your medical insurance.

What kinds of procedures does it cover? Just as important, what doesn't it cover? Does it make some options too expensive? Does it cover births at the hospitals or birth centers you're looking at?

I'd never suggest that financial criteria are the only ones that count. But you don't want to go for a form of childbirth that will leave you holding your new baby—and a fistful of unexpected medical bills. So find out which hospitals or birth centers in your area accept your insurance. Learn how many days in the hospital your policy allows for both vaginal and cesarean births. Check the specific complications your plan covers. This effort now could save you a lot of worry later on.

In the event you do not have medical insurance, it would be best to itemize (with the help of the doctor, hospital, and all involved) all possible expenses. Also, inquire about expenses for cesarean and other possibilities. With this information, you can investigate means for borrowing money in advance of its need.

The Choice Is Yours

There are two basic approaches to childbirth: natural and . . . well, not so natural, so I'll call it high-tech. That's the kind where they use machines beyond most people's ability to imagine.

The natural approach just says no to the routine use of drugs or medical procedures. It allows labor and delivery to proceed without intervention unless the safety of your wife or baby is endangered. The high-tech style uses advanced technical procedures and devices to maximize the safety and comfort of mother and child.

How does your wife feel? She might have strong feelings about what sort of birth experience she wants. Does she want to experience and feel all aspects of childbirth or would she rather do what it takes to minimize discomfort? Will she feel cheated if birth isn't as close to natural as possible? Will you?

Beyond "nature vs. technology," there are several other options. Will an obstetrician deliver your baby, or will a nurse midwife, a lay midwife, or a family practitioner?

Will your child be born at home, in the hospital delivery room, or in an alternative birth center? (Let's hope it's not on your way to the hospital!) Such centers may or may not be physically within a hospital.

Finally, there are options on the use of drugs and different procedures, as well as on the presence of husbands, birth coaches, or even other children. Before you give in to "paralysis by analysis," let's look at these who and where questions. We'll save the "what" discussion for our look at labor and delivery (see chapter IX).

It's always smart to talk to friends who are new parents. They can recommend doctors, hospitals, and procedures either to seek out or avoid. There's no more personal experience than childbirth, yet I found many people eager to talk about it, if given the chance.

Obstetrician? Midwife? Other?

Your primary practitioner isn't going to fly through the window and inform you that he or she has arrived and you can just sit back and cruise into fatherhood. And you're not going to find your doctor's name carved on the wall in the executive restroom.

Here's a good place to apply your active approach to pregnancy. That could mean reading up on childbirth and talking with your family doctor and your wife's gynecologist. Her gynecologist might be a strong candidate to deliver your baby or be able to recommend someone once he or she understands your needs.

Remember, your goal is to find a practitioner who

Many organizations provide information on pregnancy and childbirth. Here are a few:

American Academy of Pediatrics
141 Northwest Point Blvd.
Elk Grove Village, IL 60007

American College of Nurse Midwives
1522 K Street N.W., Suite 1000
Washington, DC 20005

American College of Obstetricians and Gynecologists
409 12th Street SW
Washington, DC 20024-2188

American Red Cross
17th & D Streets
Washington, DC 20006

International Childbirth Education Association (ICEA)
P.O. Box 20048
Minneapolis, MN 55420

Maternity Center Association, Inc.
48 E. 92nd Street
New York, NY 10128

makes you and your wife feel comfortable and confident. In recent years the choices a woman has in choosing her medical team have expanded. As the grip of the medical establishment upon childbirth has loosened, midwives and family practitioners have grown in prominence.

I'm (barely) old enough to remember when it wasn't that way. In the past, midwives and other nontraditional birth supervisors created an image of people engaging in obscure rituals and strange practices. But time has moved alternative birth methods into the mainstream, and this outdated image is changing.

Obstetricians and family practitioners are licensed physicians qualified to supervise childbirth. They're more likely to deliver in a hospital and favor the advantages of a high-tech approach.

These doctors are generally well equipped to handle unexpected twists in labor and delivery, and that can contribute to your sense of security. Believe me, you're going to want every bit of skill and experience your medical team can "bring to the party" during labor and delivery. If your wife has had an eventful medical history or difficulties in early pregnancy, an obstetrician is probably your best choice. The lower-risk your pregnancy, the more suitable such options as home birth or delivery by midwife become.

For some men the term "midwife" conjures up an image of a more primitive approach to childbirth, but an experienced midwife is perfectly capable of supervising most deliveries. In addition, midwives offer the advantage of continuity of care. She is not only available for your delivery but also there after the birth to assist you with your early needs. In some hospitals, your doctor may be part of a group of doctors. Any one of them could be on call when your wife will need him or her most. So there's a slight chance that the doctor with whom you've developed a good working relationship won't be around at those key moments of labor and delivery. (It's usually possible, of course, for the hospital to contact your doctor.)

There are two types of midwives: nurse and lay. A nurse midwife is a registered nurse who specializes in normal pregnancies. A lay midwife offers no such certification, and here's where you want to be very careful. Family practice physicians can treat a wide variety of conditions; their expertise is broad and it usually covers childbirth, but they aren't specialists. They are often affiliated with hospitals that offer what's called family-centered care, a medical discipline that blends sound medical practice with some nineties marketing. If your wife's pregnancy is low-risk, a family practice physician is a good middle ground choice.

The Interview

Once you have a good sense of your options in childbirth, and have tapped the "grapevine" of friends and acquaintances for prospects, it's probably a good idea to meet with the candidates.

As in most interviews, what doesn't get said is as crucial as what does. Does this person inspire confidence and trust? Does he or she have a wide range of experience in delivering babies? Does he or she have good answers to questions like:

- **What options for childbirth do you offer?**
- **Do you and the hospital allow family members or birth coaches to attend delivery?**
- **Which medications do you normally use during labor and delivery?**
- **Are you part of a group practice? If so, will you be sure to be available when my wife is due?**
- **What resources and experience do you have for complications in labor and delivery?**
- **What percentage of your deliveries are cesarean?**

You'll probably have many other questions; ask them. No question is dumb when you're pregnant. Knowledge is power, and you and your wife have every right to know.

Giving Birth at Home

Here's the ultimate in involvement for fathers-to-be. Of the 1 percent of the population who have their children at home, many do it for spiritual or philosophical reasons. There can be practical advantages as well. You might feel more comfortable at home than even in the most accommodating hospital or birth center. This can also be the way to go if you're very control conscious; nothing puts you and your wife more in control of everything that's going on. It's also a way to avoid intrusive medical procedures.

Having the degree of control that home birth gives you also means bigger responsibilities. If you're ready to consider having your baby in the friendly confines of home, a good first step is to have your wife's prenatal exam done by an obstetrician (see chapter XI). This will help you determine whether she's a good candidate for home birth. If she is, you can start looking for a midwife to be your primary caregiver during pregnancy and your main birth attendant at delivery.

Is home birth riskier than the hospital? Yes. If your wife has an eventful medical history and is having a tough pregnancy, home birth can be riskier than being in a hospital. Anyone considering home birth has to have a contingency plan for getting to a hospital in case of complications. This means that you will want to make arrangements with a hospital well in advance.

Nobody knows that better than two of my friends. Charter members of the Retired Hippies Union, not even the passage of two decades had reduced their determination to make their child's birth a cosmic experience for all.

They did their homework, made arrangements with a midwife, and worked hard to get themselves and their home ready for the big day. Unfortunately, labor wasn't exactly textbook perfect. It became apparent very quickly that help was needed that the midwife wasn't used to providing. Thankfully, the midwife knew her limitations, and they were able to get to the hospital in time.

How Will Your Home Change?

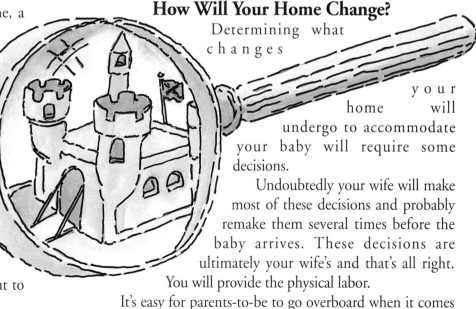

Determining what changes your home will undergo to accommodate your baby will require some decisions.

Undoubtedly your wife will make most of these decisions and probably remake them several times before the baby arrives. These decisions are ultimately your wife's and that's all right. You will provide the physical labor.

It's easy for parents-to-be to go overboard when it comes

to their living quarters—decorating every nook and cranny for baby. I'll try to spare you that expense and aggravation by putting into perspective what a newborn needs; beyond that, you're on your own.

First, your newborn will need less room than you imagine. Of course, he or she has to have a place to sleep in a bassinet and then a crib, and you will need room for clothes and supplies. But unless you're already living in a closet, you probably don't need to add that new wing to your house quite yet. It's smarter to put off a major remodel until you're well adjusted as parents.

So take a look at your house and figure out where your child can sleep (you hope). I recommend that your baby should have his or her own room. It's just a matter of time when. Whether it's two weeks or six months—the decision is yours. Whatever makes both of you feel most comfortable.

Clean out those closets whose contents you haven't touched in ages, and reserve them for clothes and small toys. And don't put off that closet-cleaning too long—do it while your wife can still help out. But do it after the two of you have talked about what items you want to keep and what can be given away or thrown out. Invariably, your ideas on this will differ. Also do it before your wife starts nesting. Haven't heard about nesting? You'll know your wife is doing it when you find her rearranging furniture, cleaning floors or carpets, or painting. Nothing unusual about that, you might say. And there isn't—unless she's doing it at two in the morning. That's nesting.

Child Proofing

One of the most important things you can do to protect your child is to make safety improvements to your home. Often we take for granted that our homes are safe, and they usually are, for adults.

But that newborn will soon be crawling and exploring areas of your home you forgot even existed. Your child will challenge you to anticipate his or her next move. "What can my child possibly get into next?" you'll ask. And you'll need to ask yourself this question repeatedly but before your child's arrival. Then you can make the necessary changes to child-proof your home.

Remember children want to taste everything as they grow. Exploring is their way of developing their motor and sensory skills and satisfying curiosity. Pay particular attention to your child's safety when you visit a house without small children, for theirs is a potential danger zone.

These are many of the home improvements you may want to do now as you're setting up your child's room. Then you will be prepared for the day (that will be here sooner than you can imagine) when your child is less dependent on you for mobility but still totally dependent on you for safety.

Toys 'R' You

I've known parents-to-be who loaded up on toys long before their children were born. It's an admirable impulse, and there's nothing wrong with picking up a few things you can't resist. But there will be plenty of time to spend major

Once your child becomes mobile you will need to have done at least the following:

• Store all under-the-sink chemicals and medicine out of reach (barely within your reach) or install cabinet locks.

• Install locks on drawers that contain utensils or sharp objects, or even tiny objects that can be easily swallowed.

• Be aware of sharp corners on tables and other furniture.

• Pay attention to drape and appliance cords that could entangle your infant.

• Place safety caps on all plugs and outlets.

• Do not leave spare change or other objects that your child can reach lying around, for they will undoubtedly be swallowed.

• Remove house plants that are poisonous.

• Use safety gates to block stairs and close off rooms or areas that your child shouldn't explore.

• Apply these cautions to your entire house and garage.

money on toys—and you'll have a much higher percentage of "hits" when you know what your child actually enjoys. So, wait and see what kinds of toys he or she likes.

You may have wondered about the "right" kinds of toys for your child. Studies show that children benefit the most, particularly in their first year, from toys that stimulate the senses, hold his or her attention, encourage interactive play, and don't pose any physical danger. But the idea that the most complicated patterns and wildest colors do your child the most good in the early months isn't the case. Simpler, high-contrast black and white geometric patterns and shapes are effective at promoting the development of motor and sensory skills.

One-on-One

Beyond toys as a developmental stimulus, I believe that the best thing a parent can do is read to his or her child, early and often. Reading is a great way to fuel a child's imagination, sense of wonder, and love of learning. Kids love stories, and they love the close "one-on-one" attention and contact that stories before bedtime bring them.

As an infant, your child will benefit from the sound and tone of your voice. As your child grows, this story time will develop into a communication time where each of you will share events from your day, questions, and concerns. Take this time to develop this rapport early with your child.

Chapter Four

A Growing Sense of Fatherhood

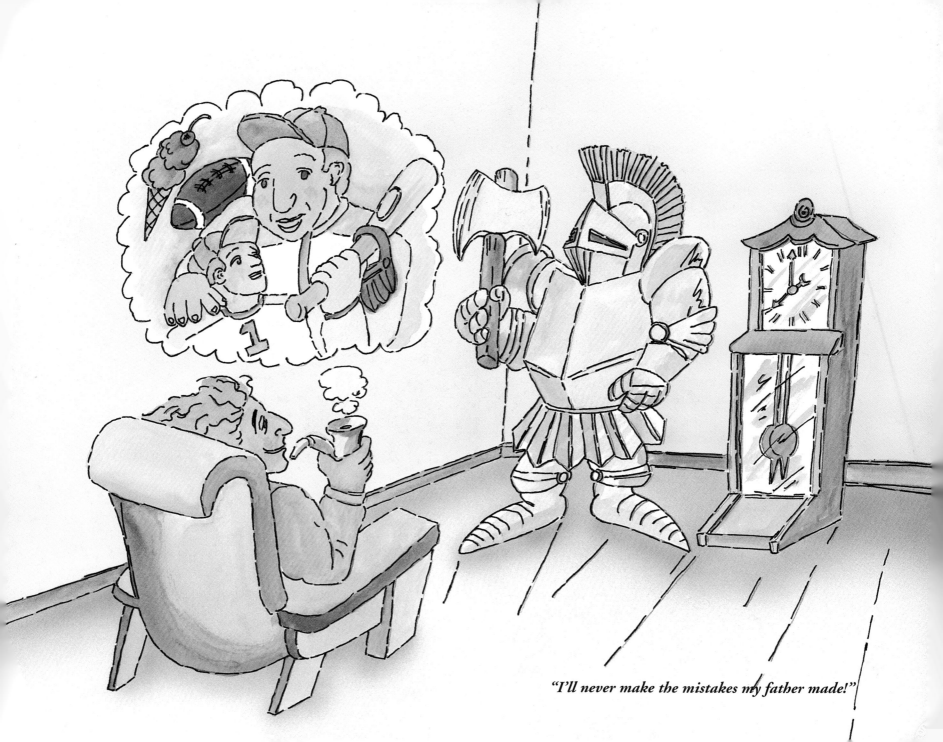

"I'll never make the mistakes my father made!"

There's a part of pregnancy that's yours and yours alone. It's what I call the "inner journey" of pregnancy—the psychological and emotional adjustment you make over thirteen months (and beyond) in which you become a father. In my case, this part of pregnancy began with memories.

Almost immediately after my wife and I got our great news, all kinds of memories of my own childhood came flooding back to me. As far as I could tell, nothing had happened to spark these recollections. But there I was in my mind's eye, five years old, trying to shovel snow off the driveway so I could shoot baskets. (Only later did I realize that my father had put up the basket to get me to do that shoveling!)

Later I found out that many men have this experience. No matter what sort of relationship you've had with your father, it's perfectly normal to have these memories. They signal the start of this inner journey to becoming a father.

If your father is alive and accessible, you might want to share some of what you're remembering with him. (You're not looking for any really deep Freudian explanation here, just doing some up-to-the-minute relating with your father.) The chances are good that the news

Emotional Scale

that he'll soon be a grandfather has sparked some reactions in him, too. There are parallels between becoming a parent and a grandparent, especially if it's the first time. Both of you are required to develop new identities, roles, and priorities.

If for any reason your father isn't around, you might want to seek out people who can help you share this inner journey. Maybe it's an associate at work who became a father recently. Maybe it's that high school or college friend you ran into and have been meaning to call.

It's reassuring to learn that what you're feeling about becoming a father— the hopes, the joys, the uncertainties, the whole package—is completely normal. That reassurance can be yours for the asking. These are some of the benefits of having family and friends.

Great Expectations . . . and Reality

When I first started seeing my child-to-be in my mind's eye, I pictured a child of about two years old who was a borderline genius, athletic, musical, and good-looking (by the way this is how many men envision their baby). This was also a child who never cried, slept through every night, never spit up, and preferred broccoli to candy. Okay, maybe my expectations were a little high.

A big factor in the inner journey during pregnancy—the psychological growth to your new identity as a father—is your expectations. Your view of how successful you are at work or on the tennis court depends a great deal on how well you meet your own, and other's, expectations.

The same applies to parenting. It's practically universal for parents-to-be to express their determination to be "perfect parents." They're intent on having all the techniques down pat and being fully versed in the latest research on children and how they develop. They tell themselves they'll remember the mistakes their parents made and will never, ever make them.

Fortunately for you, your wife, your child, and the world at large, that's a goal you won't attain. I realized this the first time I heard myself use the line, "Because I said so." That's a universal phrase guaranteed to baffle and confuse any child, any time.

Since you're going to act this way anyway, you'll be ahead of the game if you tune your expectations to match these realities. Keeping your expectations realistic, for yourself, your partner, and your child, is the cornerstone of your positive self-image as a father. It makes sense to start calibrating those expectations early in pregnancy. When you do that, you've begun to master the inner journey of pregnancy.

Without knowing you at all, I'll predict with confidence how you'll act as a parent:

• You will do the vast majority of things "right" the first time; the "mistakes" you make will be in small things and will have virtually no short or long-term effects upon your child.

• You will say and do a surprising number of things exactly the way your own father and mother did them. When you see yourself behaving this way, you'll notice it immediately, shake your head in bemused wonder, and keep right on doing them.

What to Expect of Your Wife

If it's important to keep expectations of yourself realistic, it's just as crucial to do the same for your wife.

Some people, mostly men, believe that there's something called the "maternal instinct." This instinct gives women special powers ranging from a natural aptitude for parenting to a complete set of fully refined mothering skills.

There is no scientific proof of these instincts. But, it seems that women have a greater aptitude for parenting than men. What is actually the case is women, traditionally, may have had more exposure to children. They have had more opportunities to develop those nurturing qualities. Fathers, on the other hand, have those same qualities lying dormant or undeveloped in comparison to women.

But, overall, you shouldn't assume that your wife is ahead of you in parenting skills or confidence. In fact, during pregnancy she's likely to experience many of the same doubts and apprehensions about being a parent that you might go through—as well as some that are hers alone.

Assuming that you and your wife are starting off on the same foot makes it easier to talk through those feelings. It also makes it easier for you to support each other as you move through this crash course in pregnancy and parenting.

So while you're keeping your expectations of yourself realistic, do the same for your wife. You will both benefit.

The Learning Never Stops

You've heard the expressions: "A truly wise man knows how little he really knows" . . . "The more you know, the more there is to know," and so on.

Those ideas apply directly to pregnancy and parenting. It's a lifelong learning course if there ever was one. Getting comfortable with this reality is a key adjustment you can start working on anytime during pregnancy.

Don't get me wrong—there's plenty you can learn before your baby arrives: from books, your friends and family, and your doctor. But there's only so much that you and your wife will learn that way. The real training is on the job, and you shouldn't put pressure on yourself or your wife to become

masters of parenting. Parenting is a dynamic job changing with the challenges of children. Just when you think you have it mastered, the children grow and the skills required must be revised.

I remember hearing about this from friends who became parents before my wife and I. They would talk about how fast their children were growing up and how quickly the time had passed since their children were born.

Before I became a father I discounted these remarks as comments I thought were typical of new parents. After my first child was born, I realized exactly what they meant.

You'll be dealing with a "new" child about every three months for the first two years, and the changes don't slow down much after that. Your child is constantly learning new things, developing physical skills, testing himself or herself, testing you and your wife, and challenging the world in general. This is all part of the learning and growing process.

So prepare yourself for the long haul. Look on the bright side of this adventure. You'll discover there are always new things to learn and adjust to as a parent. Along with those changes come joyous surprises and unforgettable moments that make parenting one of life's greatest experiences.

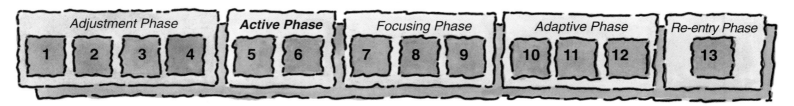

Adjustment Phase				Active Phase		Focusing Phase			Adaptive Phase			Re-entry Phase
1	2	3	4	5	6	7	8	9	10	11	12	13

The "Active" Phase

In the fifth or sixth month of pregnancy (chapters V and VI), something will happen that will change you forever. That's when your child starts moving around enough for Mom first, and then Dad, to feel it.

Lots of men can tell you the exact time, date, and circumstances when they first felt their babies move. I can recall that very moment. It's unique and special. You won't forget it either.

Feeling our child move turned the idea of becoming a father into a reality in those few moments.

For many men, questions about what kind of father they'll be and whether they truly want to be fathers, take on new urgency when they feel their babies move for the first time.

Fortunately, you'll probably have a bit more energy to deal with those questions about now. In the fifth and sixth months, the bumps are behind you and your wife. Morning sickness, if it ever arrived, is most likely over. The initial shock of learning you're pregnant is past; you're getting more comfortable with the idea and your changing identity. Worry over miscarriage recedes, and labor and delivery are still far

away. And for some couples, the middle months could be titled "the return of sex." This is partly due to your wife's renewed energy during these months. This is the same energy that drives your wife to achieve her long list of tasks and projects.

But this period also has its downside. When we weren't "oohing" and "aahing" after feeling the baby move, my wife seemed distant. I was more worried than before about my wife's and child's safety. As the reality of pregnancy became inescapable, I felt—for the first time—a closeness to my child as my connection with my wife faded to a memory.

The "Active Phase" is also when your child grows most. In these months, the typical baby will grow from two to twelve inches long; his or her weight will increase from about an ounce to a pound and a half. At the beginning of this phase, all your baby's internal organs are formed and functioning. Before the next phase starts, his or her reproductive organs become visible and your baby hears for the first time.

Chapter Five

Coping with Changes

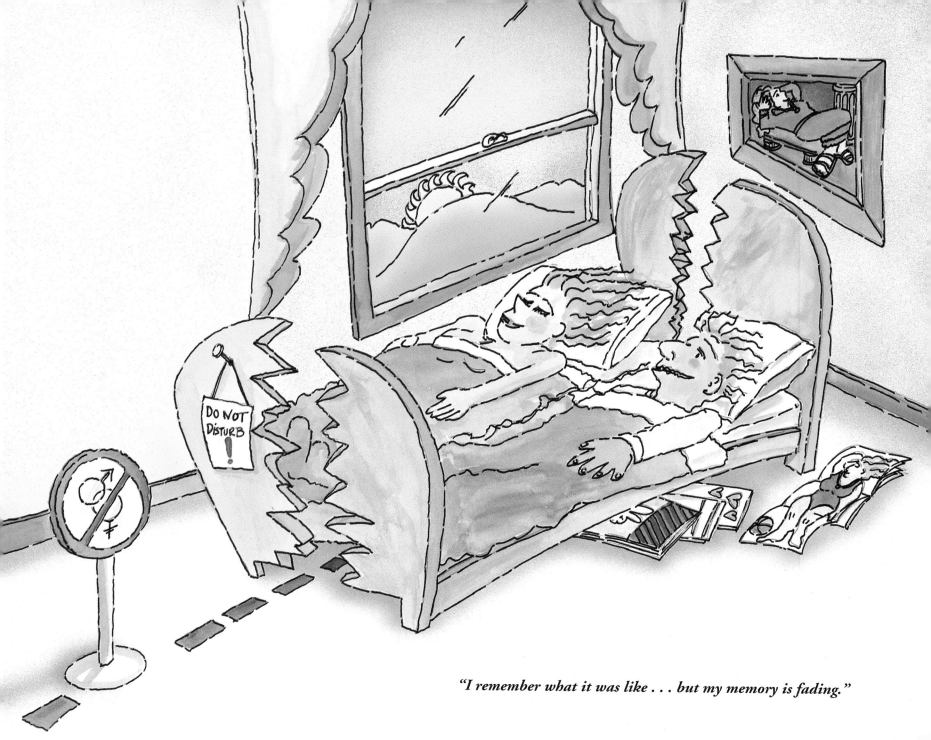

"*I remember what it was like . . . but my memory is fading.*"

You've heard the stories: insatiable women urging on dog-tired men to new feats of sexual stamina. An entire mythology has developed around sexual activity during the middle months. Like lots of myths, the notion of the sex-crazed woman contains a kernel of truth, but the full story is more complicated. When Masters and Johnson studied sex during pregnancy, 80 percent of their female respondents reported better sexual relations during the middle of their pregnancy than at the beginning. Other studies have shown that the percentages of women reporting greater, reduced, or unchanged levels of sexual interest were about equal.

While your wife's enthusiasm might normally spark your own passion, other factors could dampen your flame. If you're feeling a bit distant from your wife as she bonds with the child, if the reality of pregnancy is reviving some ambivalence within you, or if your wife's changing figure is less than a total turn-on, sex might not be at the top of your list. That's okay. No law says your sexual interest has to track perfectly with your wife's.

Some couples, though, are perfectly in sync, and they're propelled through the middle months by renewed sexual energy. For others, just the opposite is true. Some men are perplexed seeing their wives for the first time "pregnant" and have mixed feelings. My advice? Be careful!

The more your wife "shows," the more sensitive she's likely to be about how she looks. Even some innocent (or so you might think) remarks can get pounced on by a mom-to-be who is struggling to adapt to her ever-changing body.

Between You and the Mother-to-Be

It's only natural for the desire to protect your baby and partner to intensify after you've felt your baby move. That can be ironic and frustrating if you're seeing your wife and baby bond strongly with each other—and move further away from you.

Until the fourth, fifth, and sixth month, the potential dangers of pregnancy and childbirth are abstract for most men—and therefore they aren't likely to get a lot of your attention. But when you've felt your baby move and your wife is visibly pregnant, those concerns can become more real.

You might want to keep a few things in mind. First, the actual potential for harm to your wife and child is no greater—and probably less—than it's been to this point. Second, the best way to ensure the safety of Mom and child is still to use good common sense, follow your practitioner's advice, and help your partner stay well nourished and rested. (You also need to follow this advice.) And as always, expressing your fears, sharing them with your wife or doctor or a good friend, can help keep you relaxed and focused.

There are other steps you can take. I used to call my wife during the day for no particular reason. You could start up an exercise regimen, evaluate the merits of your diet, or pick a less-than-health-enhancing habit that you've wanted to break and make breaking it a top priority. Ask your doctor specific questions you have about your partner's and child's safety—no matter how "ridiculous" those questions might seem.

Advice Overload

A friend of mine told me a story about how willing people are to share their knowledge of pregnancy and children with parents-in-training.

He was walking off the basketball court after his latest failed attempt to recapture former glory. Worse yet, his team had taken another beating.

In the stands he could vaguely make out the outlines of the referee chatting with his wife and peering intently at her stomach. As he got closer he could see that the ref was moving his hand gently around her stomach.

"It's a girl," the ref said, "No doubt about it, you're going to have a girl."

"How can you tell?" his wife asked. My friend was figuring that if this guy's skill as a basketball ref was any clue, they were sure to have a boy.

"I've got the touch," he said without hesitation. "I can tell from the way you're carrying the baby. That's a little girl in there."

Five months later, when his son was born, my friend couldn't help but remember that ref.

Talking to people about pregnancy, for all its benefits, can have drawbacks. During the middle months, as your wife starts to "show," advice overload becomes an issue.

That's because the world is full of well-meaning folks, like that referee, who can't resist offering advice on pregnancy, childbirth, and parenting. Balanced skepticism is a good approach. You should be skeptical about advice (especially of the unsolicited kind) whether you're pregnant or not; that goes double for parents-to-be.

But you shouldn't dismiss any advice out of hand; that's where balance comes in. It's impossible to predict where a really valuable insight will come from, so keep yourself open to the flash of light from a source you never would have anticipated.

The fifth and sixth months promise to produce the most positive changes in your life. It is a time when much of what you have been concerned about or questioning are brought into focus and you experience closure.

Personally you will begin to feel confident in your role as a husband and as a partner in this pregnancy experience. You will feel more acceptance of your future title of father. All of these changes in attitude and feelings are the result of knowing that each of you is capable of handling your evolving roles. Also recognizing the pregnancy is well established shifts your attention to the reality that soon you will be a family.

By this time you are past the initial fanfare of your announcement. You have made the necessary adjustments at work, established a workable budget, and have some concept of how your home will look. Often men experience a calm that comes from the relief of having most of their initial questions answered and seeing the results of their organizational efforts.

By this time your wife is feeling better both physically and emotionally and can give you some much needed attention. She is often ready to listen to you regarding your career, thoughts about the upcoming event, ideas for resuming a couple's relationship, and your priorities for yourself and the family.

I found this to be one of the best times to resume "dating my wife." She had the energy and the desire (maybe even the need) to be seen as a woman first and a mother-to-be second. Just possibly she has had enough talk about "baby" (but I doubt it), that she too needs a break. She probably, like yourself, could welcome some stimulating non-baby conversation. This is often a time when your wife will recognize your sincere involvement in this whole experience. She will appreciate and respect you for your ability to balance all of these changes.

Bonding Exercises

If you and your wife seem to be "stuck" in your relationship, and are yearning to develop intimacy and grow emotionally (or are just looking for a good time that won't involve baby talk), then read on. . . .

• Visit a museum or art gallery.

• Roam around a used book store for a few hours.

• Take a drive to a secluded spot and have a picnic of your favorite delicacies.

• See a foreign film on the spur of the moment.

• Write each other love letters and poetry and exchange them at your favorite rendezvous.

• Start a hope chest, pregnancy journal, or photo album.

Relationship Update

This illustration depicts a family in which the child is the parents' only common focus. This can happen during pregnancy but should not go beyond that time.

One of the best things parents can do for their children is to work hard on their own relationship and individual growth. Your needs as an individual and as a couple should not disappear because of the arrival of your baby. It's unhealthy for everyone if you and your wife neglect these needs to focus 100 percent on your child. A relationship based solely on your child will eventually lead to conflict and may even fall apart.

Pregnancy is the ideal time for you to look at your future. Explore topics together that include how to raise your children, and what to expect of them. What type of plans do you have for your family? How many of these areas do you agree upon and where are your differences?

Action

There is no need to accept this type of relationship. It is not ideal for either you, your wife, or your child. The child can be a catalyst to pull each of you together initially if you feel this is all you have in common.

Begin by discussing your child-raising ideas, teaching concepts, and expectations for your child. Hopefully there is common ground here that can be built upon. Next, venture further to discuss non-baby ideas, plans as a family, as individuals, and as a couple. Work to explore these new ideas and areas together. By focusing on your future you may remember just how much you have in common as a couple.

Chapter Six

Your First Family Outing

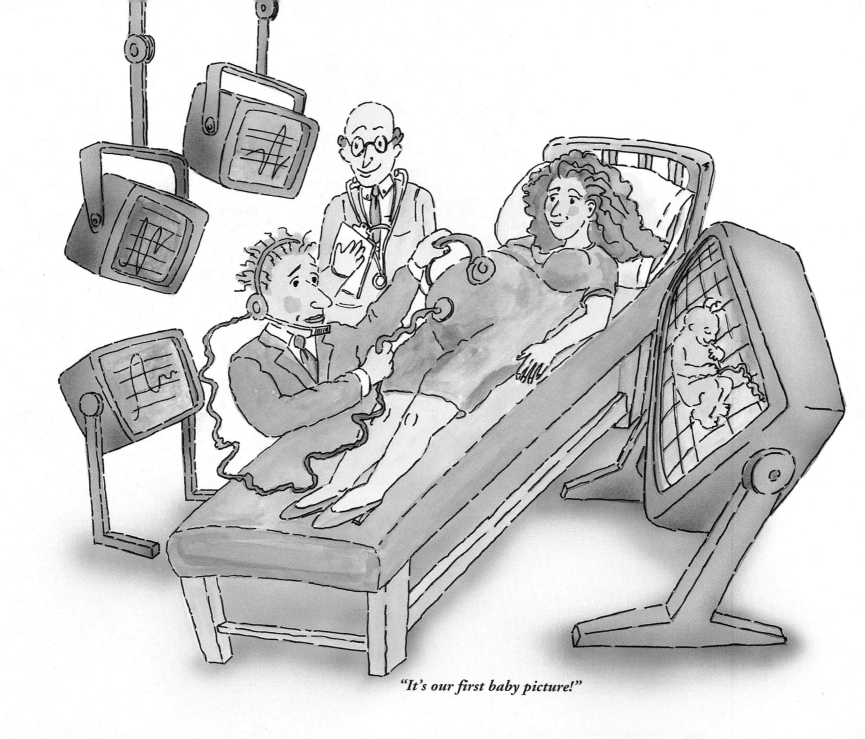

"It's our first baby picture!"

It's time for that unavoidable trip to your wife's doctor. This is one of the best ways to stay involved in your pregnancy. Assuming your wife's pregnancy is routine and low-risk, she'll be seeing her main practitioner at least fifteen times during the course of her pregnancy.

Even if you're still finalizing your "who" and "where" decisions on childbirth, your wife should make an appointment with her obstetrician/gynecologist as soon as she suspects (or knows from a home test) that she's carrying your baby. It's important to get confirmation of the pregnancy, determine when the baby is due, and get started on the regimen that will culminate in delivery.

Important, but not always easy. After she "passed" her home pregnancy test, my wife didn't hesitate to make an appointment with her obstetrician/gynecologist. "Great," I said. "Call me as soon as he's got a verdict."

"What for?" she replied. "You'll be right there with me."

"I will?" This possibility hadn't occurred to me, but I realized she was right.

Like most men, my wife's doctor wasn't much more than a name. I'd never met him or gotten within miles of his office. I certainly never intended to go along for the ride.

When the day for our first visit arrived, I was extremely nervous. I felt like I was about to enter a world where I didn't belong.

That first trip to his office didn't do much to calm my nerves. It was a doctor's office, alright, but unlike one I'd ever seen. I was surrounded by all sorts of contraptions and machines whose purposes I could probably figure out but wasn't really all that curious about. There was a noticeable shortage of sports magazines. And lots of pregnant women. I felt more self-conscious about being a man than I had since the time I accidentally wandered into the girls locker room in junior high school.

Meeting the doctor didn't help much either. He looked like a guy who could pick up some pocket money as a model in *GQ* if his main business ever slowed down. And—the ultimate insult—he was definitely younger than I was. I made a mental note to attend all future appointments.

But my wife and I survived that visit, and after becoming a regular at these pregnancy checkups, I grew to like and respect the doctor. I realized soon enough that his interest in my wife's most private bodily parts and functions was strictly clinical.

The goal of this first visit is to give your doctor the information he or she needs to determine whether your wife's pregnancy is likely to be routine. To make this determination, the doctor will gather information on your wife's medical history (and some about yours), give her a thorough physical examination, and perform the first in a series of tests that will enable all of you to track the development of your child.

Medical History

No surprises here. Do you, your wife, or either of your immediate family members have any present health problems or "medical skeletons" that might affect the pregnancy? If so, now is the time to talk about them. Your doctor will go through a long list of questions about things like allergies, chronic illnesses or conditions, any prescription medicines you or your wife are taking, and more; you shouldn't hold anything back.

Physical Exam

The basics of a physical don't change when you're pregnant; what's added is the doctor's examination of your wife's pelvis to determine its "fitness" for delivery. The doctor will also check your wife's uterus, since its size correlates roughly with the age of the baby. Finally, your wife will have a standard vaginal exam, including a Pap smear as a check for cervical cancer and a manual examination of her ovaries.

Test Time

The initial workup also includes a blood sample to see whether your wife is anemic and to make sure there's no risk of incompatibility between Mom and child when it comes to their blood types, which can cause problems. Blood screening will also make sure your wife has the right antibodies in the right quantities (primarily the rubella antibody) and none of the wrong ones.

In addition, the doctor will take a urine sample to run a glucose test that checks for gestational diabetes, an odd temporary condition that sometimes sets in because the effectiveness of insulin (for some mysterious reason) decreases during pregnancy. He or she will also take a culture to look for kidney or bladder infections.

You may be surprised at how many tests your wife goes through in this first visit, but think about it: There's a new life growing within her and the adjustments her body is making are profound. Tests that monitor those changes make good sense.

If you're like some people I know, you might be thinking at this point, "Oh, yeah, it's really great what they can do in checking out the baby for all this stuff, but . . . you know me, I'm one of those guys who'd rather not know . . . what you don't know won't hurt you, right?" But that's an outdated approach, isn't it? In the information age of the nineties, we have the opportunity to reduce the potential for surprises by arming ourselves with essential knowledge. That's what these tests offer.

The following are the most common tests performed during the fourth, fifth, and sixth months. The purpose of these tests is to make sure there are no serious defects or abnormalities, as well as to hone in on the age of your baby. Consult your doctor for the details and risks involved.

Ultrasound (Your first baby pictures!):

Purpose—Stage 1 ultrasound can discern the baby's heart rate, its age, position of placenta, and confirm diagnosis of twins. (Ready to "double your pleasure," Dad?) Stage 2 ultrasound is used to determine presence of congenital defects.

Timing—First scan at three to four months, others can be done at any time later in pregnancy.

Procedure—Usually done in the doctor's office (or at the hospital) by applying sound waves to the mothers abdomen. This test is exciting for both of you. You may be able to determine your child's sex, which a lot of parents really like. Do you want to know? Discuss it in advance, and decide.

Risks—No apparent risks documented to date.

Alpha fetoprotein (AFP) screening:

Purpose—AFP is a chemical whose higher-than-normal presence in mother's blood sometimes indicates neural tube defects, which are abnormalities of the spine or brain such as spina bifida. High number of false positives; AFP levels can also be higher when carrying twins, so the doctor will follow up any questionable results with amniocentesis.

Timing—Fourth to fifth months.

Procedure—Blood test.

Risks—None.

Amniocentesis:

Purpose—To uncover birth defects, including Down's syndrome and spina bifida.

Timing—Fourth to fifth months; for all women over thirty-five, or if your wife carries genetically linked disorders such as hemophilia.

Procedure—It is normally conducted at the hospital on an "outpatient" basis.

Risks—Low.

Pain Relief

Helping your wife deal with the discomfort that often (but not always) occurs in labor and delivery is the biggest contribution you can make. The question is, Dad—want some help?

Modern medicine offers three kinds of pain relievers: analgesics (which numb the pain center in the brain), anesthetics (which dull sensation), and tranquilizers (which make one sleepy).

The issue for you and your wife to decide, well before labor begins, is how you both (but especially your wife) feel about using pain relievers. Some women, especially with their first children, want to experience childbirth without any help; others are just as eager to minimize discomfort. It's not a "moral" issue, either. She's not a better woman if she decides to forego pain relief.

One thing to consider is the potential effect of pain relievers on your baby and wife. Some tranquilizers sedate your baby for several days. Others can extend labor. Check with your practitioner; ask him or her to review the options and potential side effects.

What sometimes happens is that women go into labor having decided to skip pain relievers, only to feel differently when they're in the grip of the real thing. This is something you and your wife should talk about during these months. Remind her that it's not a sign of "weakness" if she changes her mind. My wife didn't feel badly at all when she requested (actually, she demanded) a pain reliever during labor.

In recent years epidurals (administered by injection) have become popular. Many women feel this is as close to an ideal solution as exists. This form of anesthetic helps relieve your wife's pain but doesn't dull her awareness or, apparently, affect your baby. An epidural is essentially a local anesthetic whose effects last several hours and can be extended by readministering the anesthetic.

Again, discuss this area of pain relief early and raise any questions with your doctor.

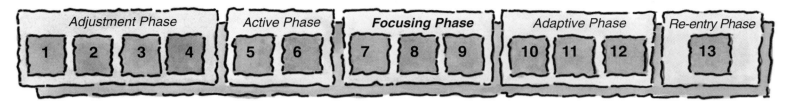

Adjustment Phase				Active Phase		Focusing Phase			Adaptive Phase			Re-entry Phase
1	2	3	4	5	6	7	8	9	10	11	12	13

The "Focusing" Phase

There are three main themes in the seventh, eighth, and ninth months (chapters VII-IX): preparation, preparation, and more preparation.

Everything you do during these months is geared toward getting you and your wife ready for labor and delivery. If you find yourselves too involved in tasks that aren't helping you prepare, step back for a minute. This may not be the best time to work on your antique car collection or refinish those hardwood floors. Of course, these activities either help you relax (a big part of preparation) or help you keep your job (a big part of being able to relax).

Many couples find that everything about pregnancy seems to intensify during the home stretch. Feelings or issues appear to take on more urgency and time seems shorter. This is a time when the simplest remark or behavior can be blown out of proportion—by you or your wife. So it's important for both of you to make allowances and be especially flexible as childbirth draws near.

I'll never forget the day at the start of our seventh month. It had been a typical pressure cooker at work, and I was looking forward to an unhurried evening at home.

So you can imagine my surprise when I went to open the door and heard my wife screaming as loudly as she could. I froze. What was going on?

I opened the door cautiously. The screaming stopped and my wife emerged from the back room. "Hi, honey," she said as if nothing had happened. "How was your day?"

Now I was totally confused. "What was that all about?" I said, half panicked and half angry. "Oh, that was nothing," she said. "I just figured a little screaming was a good way to work off some of the stress." Pregnancy is full of firsts!

During these months, your stress level is likely to rise as well. Your wife's physical discomfort is at its peak, which, along with her apprehension over labor and delivery, can make it harder for her to sleep well. (And if she can't sleep, don't be too surprised if she wants you to stay up and keep her company.) In addition, your wife is going to need more help than ever from you with tasks around the house. This, on top of your nervousness over labor and delivery, can make you more irritable.

You may also be feeling a sharper rivalry between you and your new baby. As your wife gets tired more easily, and less able to "carry her weight" around the house, it's easy for you to feel put-upon by this baby you haven't even met yet. But look at the bright side. You're getting ready for birth and early fatherhood. I got plenty of practice at washing dishes, vacuuming, and doing the laundry that would come in handy later on.

I can almost hear you say, "Who needs to practice that stuff? What I need is some time to myself. Why didn't they tell me that pregnancy would last forever?" I remember those feelings well. I will remind you that there's more of pregnancy behind you than in front of you; your patience and stamina are about to be rewarded with a son or daughter.

You may also be feeling a bit frustrated if, as can happen, the level and ease of sexual intimacy in your marriage drops off sharply. The key to dealing with these feelings is to recognize first that they're completely normal and short-lived. I was a little slow to learn. I collected two speeding tickets attempting to grind my frustration into the road.

Remember too that these months aren't all bleak. You might experience a surge of energy at work and at home, contrary to how your wife is feeling. Impending fatherhood (and its inescapable increased responsibility) spurs you to "aim higher" at work. The imminence of birth helps lots of men focus, prioritize, and act. Finally, the last three months before birth mean the end of pregnancy is in sight.

The biggest issue during this time is your role in labor and delivery. I'll help you look at what you and your wife can do to help address this issue through participation in a childbirth class. I also offer guidelines on preparations at home and at work.

Chapter Seven
Getting Ready

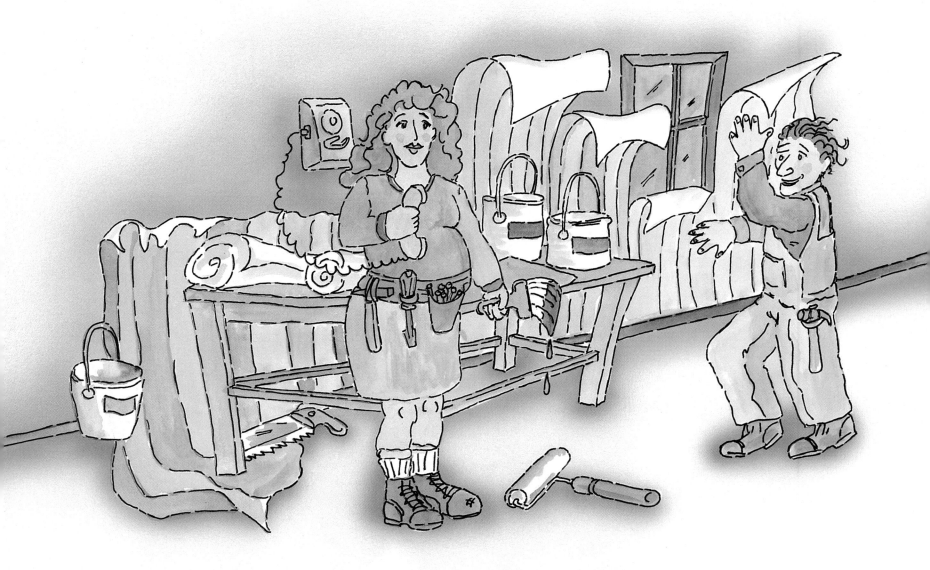

"The commercials for those do-it-yourself books made it look so much easier."

Are you still rearranging or even remodeling? I suggested postponing that huge remodeling job in favor of less drastic preparations. In my pregnancy, I decided to do the renovations that I'd always intended to get to but hadn't yet. Learning I was going to be a father was the spark I needed, and soon my nights and weekends (when I was at home, that is) were spent remodeling the house.

I set up a schedule so that everything would get done about a week before our baby was due. Before I knew it, I was behind schedule. I finally called in some professional help, and we finished up the day before our daughter was born. It's a good thing she arrived two weeks late!

Now let's see how you can avoid that sort of mad scrambling around when you should be strongly focused on getting ready for childbirth. I'll never forget the time I asked a friend with two small children for advice on getting ready for the baby. I had looked forward to this person's suggestions because he'd always had sharp insights. He answered without hesitation. "Just make sure your washing machine works and that you have a freezer full of food." I was shocked. I had expected some keen and wise suggestions; six months later I realized that's exactly what I'd gotten.

The reason is simple. Once your child is born, you can't dash off to the store (or live 96 percent of your life) the way you used to. And you'll have plenty of clothes to wash!

But wait, you're saying. What do household preparations have to do with you? You're not going to become Mr. Mom as soon as your baby arrives.

No, but if you're like me you'll spend more time doing housework in your first months as a father than you've done in your whole life. And because your baby is involved, you'll probably wind up enjoying those chores more than you ever thought possible. Getting the work done with a newborn makes whatever division of labor you and your wife have set up around the house radically different. And that may mean more time in the kitchen, supermarket, and laundry room than you're probably spending now.

But that's a break for you, Dad. That kind of work is a practical, helpful outlet for the innate desire you'll have to protect, nurture, and comfort your newborn. It's also the basis for developing an early relationship with your child. It's the best possible support you can offer in the final three months before birth.

Back to Basics

A newborn's needs are actually simple: food, clothing, shelter and all the love parents can give.

"Food's no problem," I can hear you saying. "My wife's going to breast-feed. If anything gets me off the hook, that will." Maybe not, Dad. More women in the nineties are using breast pumps in order to have a ready supply of milk at hand. If your wife prefers this approach to "nursing on demand," you can be a big help in keeping the bottles clean and feeding your baby.

The advantages of breast-feeding—its nutritional value, its convenience, the emotional rewards for mother and child, the immunities it provides your baby—are clear. It's the way to go unless she's had breast surgery, taking medication that shouldn't be passed to a newborn, or returning to work within a few months. These factors would make breast-feeding impractical.

So if your child will use a bottle, you'll want to have a good supply of formula, and the equipment you need for preparing it. Bottles and nipples should be on hand all the time. But don't buy too much until you find out what kind of formula your doctor and child prefer. And whether your baby feeds at breast or bottle, there are many other ways in which you can help out. You can burp the baby or get him or her out of bed for those 2 A.M. feedings. You can be in charge of the towels that will come in handy for the inevitable spit-up that follows many feedings. It's not the most glamorous work, but my guess is that you'll learn to accept it! And besides, its over before you know it.

Supplies

Figuring out what to buy for your baby can be as exhausting as doing it; I'll just cover the basics here. My goal is to make you aware of your child's needs. There's a good chance your wife will pick up a lot of useful supplies at baby showers and as gifts after your baby is born.

In addition, this is an area that many women enjoy taking the lead; if that's the case with your wife, why stand in her way? In fact most of what follows is intended as a summary of what *is* needed. It's most likely your wife will already know this and take great pride in procuring these essential items.

There's one rule that's a constant: your baby's needs will change rapidly in the first few months, so don't go haywire on shopping quite yet. It's better to concentrate on getting well stocked with what you'll need for the first couple of weeks. You'll want plenty of those one-piece outfits that are easy to take off and put on (once you've done it about twenty times). It's more likely your wife will already know this and take great pride in procuring these items. You should have plenty of diapers on hand, either cloth or disposable, as well as some gentle wipes. Tiny undershirts, plenty of socks and booties, and a ready supply of small towels to put on your shoulder before you put your baby there as you carry him or her around, are essential.

This was another lesson I learned the hard way. One morning I was rushing out the door to a meeting as my wife finished feeding our daughter. She asked me to burp her—normally about a sixty second job—and I agreed. Rather than find a towel, I figured I'd chance it and go unprotected. It was a gamble I lost, and soon enough I was upstairs changing into another suit for the office.

Your baby's crib should have a firm mattress, and you should get several waterproof covers for it. Also make sure that the crib has padding around the sides. Pillows are not to be used in the crib. It's too easy for little ones to suffocate under them.

Blankets should be thin—quilts are out for newborns for the same reason as pillows. You'll also want to stock up on fitted sheets, which provide extra warmth if they're flannel.

A portable "spring" seat is also a handy piece of equipment. This is about the size of a child's first car seat, set at about a forty-five degree angle, that your child sits in when he or she is in the house (or in other people's houses) with you. It lets your child take in all the sights, relieves you of the burden of carrying him or her around every minute, and helps sharpen your child's developing senses. It's also handy for transporting your baby almost anywhere— the neighbor's, the market, your favorite restaurant.

After a few weeks, your stroller and diaper bag will be as familiar to you as the back of your hand. Your child will outgrow a couple of strollers in his or her first few years, so you needn't break the bank on the first one. You'll always want to be able to strap your baby into the stroller, and I'd strongly recommend one that folds up for easy storing in the car.

A diaper bag—what my wife calls our "Normandy invasion kit"—is where you keep diapers, wipes, formula if you use it, and a change of clothes (or three) for those "unexpected" emergencies you know are going to happen. You won't be going anywhere without these supplies for many months, so get a bag that's sturdy yet easy to haul around. And get one that's about twice as big as what you think you'll ever need.

You'll also want to set up a changing table somewhere in your house. This is any surface where you can place your baby to change diapers and clothes. Since this will be done many times each day, get a table that's big enough (and the correct height) to do the job easily.

A portable bath is also part of your basic setup. You can, of course, wash your newborn in the kitchen or bathroom sink. But most couples prefer a separate little bath basin for their newborns.

Your child's car seat is one of the most important purchases you'll make, but again, the most expensive one is not necessarily the best. (I wouldn't buy the least expensive one either.) You need one that doesn't require a Ph.D. in nuclear physics to use, and you'll probably want one you can wash, although you're never going to keep the seat spotless. Your child will outgrow his or her first (and probably second) car seat, and some parents may want to have a backup in the trunk or at the in-laws.

During your pregnancy you've probably noticed many parents carrying their babies in either front-loading packs and then (when they're a little older) in backpacks. These give your child a great view of all sorts of other key firsts, and free your hands up in the process.

Don't forget to stock up on birth announcement notes and little thank-you cards for the gifts you're sure to get. Of course, there will be plenty of people you'll want to notify of your blessed event by phone. My wife and I found that putting together a list of these people, with phone numbers, saved time and hassle when it came time to make those calls. It's really easy to forget phone numbers—even ones you've dialed frequently—in the moments after you become a father.

Lots of film for your camera is a good idea. Pictures are second only to videotapes as the best record of your child's growth. Pictures make more sense in the early weeks to pass along to family and friends. You'll want to take dozens, so be ready with film and several albums. (This is a great time to start keeping your pictures in albums if you don't already.) This is an area I took charge of, since I realized early I would be the family historian. The first few months of your baby's life are rich in photo opportunities—don't miss them.

There are several "flavors" of childbirth classes, derived largely from different approaches to childbirth:

• Grantly Dick-Read—The granddaddy of organized childbirth-preparation methods, Grantly Dick-Read relies on education and relaxation to move your wife successfully through labor and delivery.

• Lamaze—This approach stresses relaxation techniques to combat the pain of childbirth and provides information on how to deal with contractions during labor. *American Society for Psychoprophylaxis in Obstetrics, (ASPO Lamaze) 1101 Connecticut Ave. N.W., Washington D.C. 20036*

• Bradley—This was the first childbirth method that enlisted fathers as coaches. The Bradley approach emphasizes exercise and deep breathing; classes typically span all nine months of pregnancy. *American Academy of Husband Coached Childbirth, P.O. Box 5224, Sherman Oaks, CA 91413*

Childbirth Classes

A well-taught childbirth class can give you and your wife information, encouragement, and support. You should plan to take one during the last three months of pregnancy.

Many classes combine elements of the common and more obscure philosophies. Word-of-mouth about instructors is probably the key to finding a good class, so don't be afraid to seek out new parents and ask who they recommend. Hospitals and birth centers can also get you started by providing listings of all available classes in your area—many of which are held at those hospitals and centers.

Fathers-to-be can derive many benefits from childbirth classes. They can be great sources of useful information; the teacher usually encourages questions and the sharing of feelings and experiences with your classmates. You can take the needed reassurance home from your weekly sessions.

You've always known that you'd be a great coach if you had the chance, right? Well, childbirth classes give you that chance. Like all the great teams, you and your wife are working toward a common goal—being successful parents. You each have your jobs to do, and teamwork is the key. So think of your childbirth class as training camp for the "big game" that's coming up.

A good class can strengthen that teamwork and bond between you and your wife. It can go a long way toward calming your nerves about labor and delivery. It can bring you into contact with people who are becoming parents at the same time you are, and lots of friendships (not to mention baby-sitting-exchange arrangements) begin in childbirth classes.

In fact, your classmates can be an excellent network for you and your wife during those early months of parenthood, especially when you feel "stranded" at home. Most likely, your classmates will be going through the same thing.

Support is a very strong argument in favor of finding a good class and sticking with it. In addition to its practical benefits, my childbirth class was a nice reprieve from the stresses of work and pregnancy. It reassured me and my wife that we weren't alone; it can do the same for you.

At the Movies

I recall attending childbirth classes and waiting for the day when we would see those famous "birth" movies. You may be familiar with these already, but if not, it's something to anticipate. They are very colorful and clinical. I believe they are an attempt to expose you to the more graphical aspects of labor and delivery. They leave very little to the imagination. So when it's the real thing you'll know exactly what to expect.

If you start feeling a bit queasy, remember they present the facts and are a reasonable first-time exposure. Your actual delivery moments will unfold differently and will be emotionally and psychologically unique to you as a couple. But the physical aspects of birth will undoubtedly be a sequence from these movies.

Getting Ready at Work

Fathers-to-be often feel energized during the final months before birth, and that can help you focus and stay motivated at work. But you also might feel distracted, as your thoughts turn to the impending birth and your first few weeks as a father. It doesn't pay to worry too much if your mind wanders; didn't that happen even before you got pregnant, when a meeting would drag on too long?

There are seven proven steps you can take during this time to help you stay on top of your workload while you get ready for fatherhood. They are:

1) **Stay in close touch with your employer; make sure you understand what your priorities are and exactly what's expected of you. If you're the boss, make sure your goals and priorities are set and well known by your employees.**

2) **Resist any temptation to take on any additional or long-term projects. Concentrate on your core duties and make sure you're giving those your undivided attention.**

3) **Minimize your participation in club involvements and professional groups that take away from your time.**

4) **Try to work on projects that are team efforts; that way, when you have to "drop out" temporarily to attend to your growing family, the impact will be minimized.**

5) **Square away your arrangements for time off after your** child is born (your company may offer paternity leave). **I'd suggest that you plan on anywhere from a week to two weeks. Any less is too little time for your family to start to get its new routines established; any more and you'll probably lose your mind.**

6) **If possible, don't schedule any travel during the last month of pregnancy.**

7) **Keep reasonable hours. After your child is born, you'll probably find yourself hanging back at home as long as you can, and wanting to dash home at the stroke of five. Ease into it during these final months. Sleep whenever and wherever you can.**

Chapter Eight

Lights . . . Camera . . .

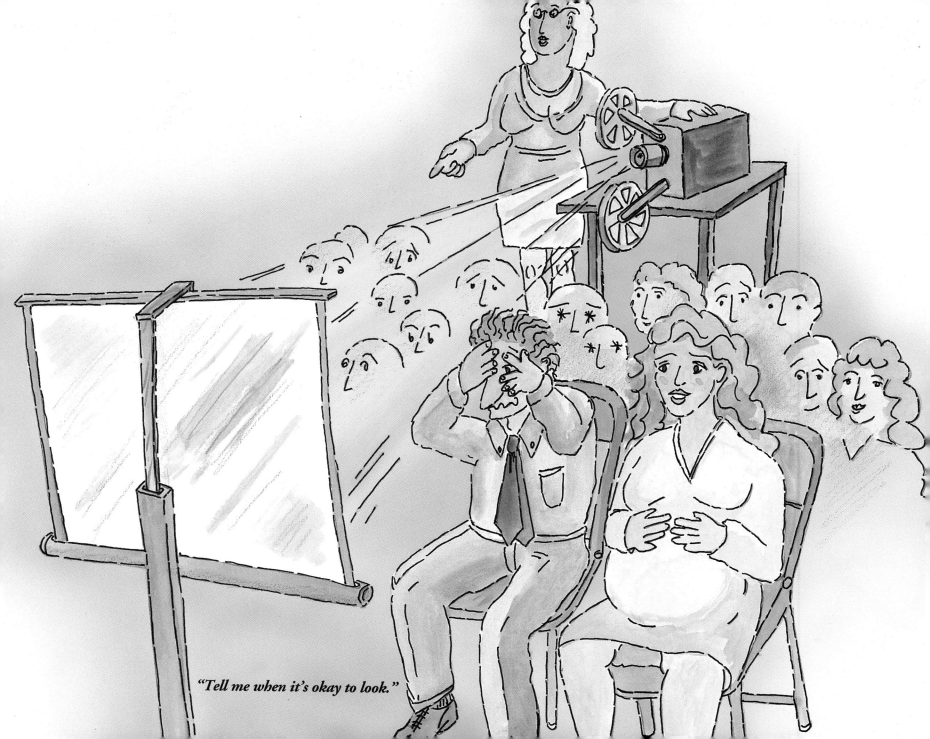

"Tell me when it's okay to look."

Consider yourself warned: the last weeks before birth can be touchy! You and your wife might be grappling with perfectly normal apprehension and excitement over what's coming up. Childbirth classes and your wife's growing physical discomfort can make it easy to obsess about labor and delivery. For you, that can raise tough questions: What role will you play in childbirth? How well will you do? Can you handle it?

Answering the first question is the best reason for taking a childbirth class. Clearly, a big factor in your success at helping your wife—and yourself—during childbirth is based upon what kind of birth you're planning. A home birth gives you a bigger role than you'll have at a hospital or birthing center, but no birth frees you, Dad, from a significant role.

Today it's not the norm for fathers to sit in the waiting room until the doctor comes out to make his announcement. That was the style of our fathers and grandfathers, but those days are way past. For the nineties man, active participation in pregnancy and childbirth makes much more sense.

That change is more than one of just style. Studies reported in the *Journal of the American Medical Association* show that a supportive companion during childbirth makes labor and delivery easier. And it's reasonable to assume that easier labor and delivery can shorten the time it will take your family to get back on track.

The best thing you can do for your wife during childbirth is to comfort and encourage her as she goes through the most challenging, mysterious, exhilarating, and

Support Basics

• Be well informed on labor and delivery. Chapter IX gives you the fundamentals, and there are plenty of other good books where you can get more detail. (That's if your wife hasn't already given you a synopsis from every one of those books piled on her nightstand.)

• Practice the breathing and relaxation techniques you're learning in class before your mad dash to the hospital. This is about all you can practice; it's not much, but when labor starts you'll be glad you did.

• Arrange a tour of your hospital or birth center so that you and your wife are familiar with labor and delivery rooms. During the most eventful hours of labor, you and your wife can become extremely sensitive to otherwise normal events in your surroundings—medical staff bustling around, equipment being moved in and out. Take time to familiarize yourself with those surroundings.

• Make an effort to get to know your classmates; what better people to share your feelings and experiences with than other novice parents?

humbling event of her life. (This assumes that she hasn't previously had children or been abducted by UFOs.)

Delivery-room *performance anxiety* is almost universal among fathers during the last weeks of pregnancy. It's easy to dream up scenes in which you're reduced to a quivering blob just when your wife (and child) need you the most. Lots of men have images of fainting after they've been panicked by the reality of the birth moment.

"But really," you ask, "who ever really worries about performance anxiety?" "I'll do just fine," I thought. "We've practiced our breathing, the movies didn't scare me, and we have a great doctor." But as time went on, my thoughts and concerns about the actual delivery occurred more frequently.

Then the day came. My wife called the office to tell me it was time to head for the hospital. I wasn't there and my assistant didn't know where I was. An hour later, I happened to call home and it was clear she was panicked. I had taken both sets of car keys and no friends were around to take her to the hospital. I raced home only to be stopped and ticketed for speeding.

Eventually, I arrived home to find my wife's contractions coming regularly. Labor had begun. I helped her into the car, forgetting her bag, and sped toward the hospital. Moments into the trip, the car ran out of gas. I jumped from the car and ran up to four houses before anyone answered. I needed desperately to call a taxi. I remember my wife saying, "Hurry, hurry, I can't wait!"

The taxi service promised ten minutes. I pleaded for five. And then we waited. By now, we were both anxious and still waiting twenty minutes later. My wife was pale and breathing irregularly as the contractions came one after the other.

The taxi finally appeared and we were again on the way to the hospital. It was about ten minutes later, when I first looked up expecting to be arriving at the hospital. It was then I realized the driver was going to the wrong hospital. At my command he swung the car around and headed for our destination.

Now my wife was talking in short spurts about delivering in the back seat. At that point, I thought, "You might as well." The traffic was stopped, I forgot to call our doctor, and the completed admission forms were safe at home. What more could go wrong? Then my wife yelled, "Hurry, it's time, it's time!" as she pulled on my arm.

It was at that moment that the alarm clock went off and I woke up from a deep sleep. My wife was gently tugging on my arm reminding me, "It's time, it's time . . . to get up." Thank God, it was only a dream.

I must have been worried about my delivery-room performance, but this dream encouraged me to get more involved in our pregnancy.

Even if you're worried now about what will take place in childbirth, whatever happens will quickly become a memory. Soon after your baby arrives, you'll be so overjoyed that you'll wonder what you were so worried about. Besides, you're already doing a lot to calm your anxiety: reading, working on teamwork with your wife, talking to friends who are parents and taking your class.

Name That Child!

Entire shelves at bookstores contain books on children's names. Many couples spend a lot of time, most of it quite pleasant, sifting through hundreds of possible names.

Be ready for your wife to spend much more time at this than you do. She may even wake you up in the middle of the night to ask your opinion on a name she's thought of. Patience, Dad, patience.

What some couples forget is that there's no law that says you have to go through weeks of profound deliberations to come up with a name. My wife and I didn't. She had a few good ideas (which was a few more than I had), we talked about them, came up with one (one of each sex) we both really liked, and we were done. I've spoken to couples who knew within seconds of completing a home pregnancy test what they wanted to name their child. If that's the case with you, don't fight it.

But there's also no problem if you don't have a clue about names. That's why there are so many books, and those books can show you the range of possibilities (if they don't confuse you first).

You and your wife might have several names you've been partial to for a long time. Start your search with those. Maybe you want to name your child after your favorite baseball player, rock and roll star, or writer. Or maybe it's that teacher or professor you remember most. And then there are family members, relatives, or friends you might want to honor in this special way.

Those are all good reasons; if you and your wife agree on the person and the name sounds good, you might have it.

Why "might"? Because practically every couple settles on a name only to discover a few days later that they haven't really settled. That's okay. There's no point in punishing yourselves for second thoughts. It's one of the few decisions in life that you can go back on without any consequences. (That is, before your baby is born!)

But it's equally pointless to put off your final decision until, say, the ride to the hospital or after the baby is born. First, it's wrong to hope that seeing your child will tell you what his or her name should be. In addition, you'll be focusing on many other things in the immediate aftermath of childbirth—there won't be much time for the cool contemplation you'll need.

And when it comes to picking a name, you can do your child a big favor before he or she is born. Avoid any temptation you might feel to give your offspring one of those "unusual" names. You've probably seen the books that list the strangest-but-true names around: Ima Hogg . . . Jim Shooz . . . Patty Cake. A friend of mine once worked with someone named Sterling Silver. Now, somebody with a name like that could have found a cure for cancer, but most people aren't able to get past the name. Studies of children with unusual names show that they're more likely to get teased as they grow up—and who teases more cruelly than kids?

And keep in mind that the popularity of different names goes in cycles. Today's trendy name is likely to be dated twenty years from now. That's why there are fewer women today named Violet or Iris than in your grandmother's generation.

Late-Pregnancy Sex

The "typical" pattern is for sex to almost vanish during the last weeks of pregnancy, but who says you have to be typical?

My wife and I were one of those couples for whom lovemaking didn't disappear, down to the home stretch. We adjusted to her growing size and her bouts of discomfort, we experimented a bit and our love life prospered.

And there is something special—beyond novelty—about being intimate during these weeks. My wife and I needed support and encouragement, and we found comfort in our lovemaking. It helped my wife's confidence in her physical desirability, and kept me feeling close to my wife.

Of course, we also had friends for whom lovemaking of any sort had become just a fond memory by the late stages of pregnancy; this is also quite common. As always, there's no right or wrong regarding sexual activity in the final weeks of pregnancy. First, your partner needs to be cleared by her doctor (and you shouldn't feel shy about asking the doctor). Second, make sure neither of you is uptight about feeling that your baby is "watching" (in fact the baby has no awareness of what's going on). Finally, if you crave the mutual tenderness and affirmation that intimacy between lovers can offer, sex should be on your to do list for the three months prior to birth.

But don't be surprised if it's on your list and not your wife's. If you've been supportive and attentive over the past few months, the chances are better that this won't happen. But it's also important for neither of you to push the other if one isn't feeling the desire to make love. Even if you're one of those men who wonders whether he'll ever make love again, a little more patience and understanding during these weeks will truly pay great dividends later on.

Your Wife Is Uncomfortable . . . a Lot

Although nothing your wife experiences during pregnancy can compare with the discomfort she's likely to endure during childbirth, get plenty of practice helping her deal with physical discomfort as your baby's arrival gets closer. What sort of discomfort? An occasional headache, dizziness, or fainting. More difficulty than usual sleeping. (This might be nature's way of getting you both ready for those 3:00 A.M. feedings.) Pain in her back, maybe swollen feet and ankles, and swings in appetite, energy, and moods.

Individually, any of these might not be much more than an inconvenience; together, they can make your wife fed up with being pregnant. "I'm so tired of being pregnant" was a complaint I heard often during this time. Well, how would you like to carry around all that extra weight for all that time? I realized later that my wife's complaints were actually cries for sympathy, and a few kind words of encouragement from me would have been greatly appreciated.

The best way for you to handle the discomforts and complaints is to deal with them promptly and cheerfully. That's not always easy; you've got to be patient, flexible, and understanding.. You're in luck—those are the qualities you'll need as a father. So think of this as good training. Of course, if any of your wife's symptoms are severe, persistent, or if she's bleeding, consult your doctor immediately.

A Common Theme

All these topics—your role in labor and delivery, helping your wife handle physical discomfort, and naming your child—have a common thread: teamwork. In fact, that's what the last three months before birth are all about: you and your wife sharpening your ability to work together to meet the challenge of becoming parents. Nothing puts a higher premium on successful teamwork than parenting.

Why? Because being parents changes your focus from yourselves to your child. That's an idea you can read about during pregnancy and perhaps accept on an intellectual level. But after your baby is born, it's something that you'll be living so deeply you'll barely notice it. I can hear your question already: "So, after my baby arrives, that means we won't be a couple again?" The short answer is . . . yes. Because if you define being a couple as being what you were before, forget it.

But here's the good news: Being parents is a chance to be a new kind of couple, different than you've ever been before. Being focused on a common goal (such as raising your child to win that Nobel Prize), and being responsible for someone beyond yourselves is one of the most exciting adventures. Parenting will show you aspects of yourselves and each other you never dreamed existed—most of which you'll be happy to discover. It will challenge you in ways you'll never anticipate. Believe it or not, you'll soon wonder why you waited so long.

You'll never again be the couple you were, but the new version will be closer and happier in ways it's hard to imagine when you're not a parent. The active role you've taken during pregnancy shows your wife that you really care about being a father. Your wife will appreciate this new dimension of your personality, just as you'll come to admire her skill as a mother.

Relationship Update

This illustration displays another situation to avoid or work to correct. Both you and your wife are doing fine in your relationship but you have removed yourself from your child's development.

Many factors can cause this to occur. Maybe you have not won your wife's full confidence in you as a father. Or you are worrying that your relationship with your wife is about to be changed in a way you won't like. Sometimes it's the thought that you're not really ready to be a father. Whatever your reasons are, you have allowed your wife to assume the role of chief child developer while you pursue your career or other interests.

A truly healthy, couple relationship, would foster the interaction of both parents with the child. The child's development depends upon a balanced approach by the parents. While the mother may be the primary caregiver, your participation helps your child feel part of a developing family.

This type of relationship requires your immediate attention for the health and well being of everyone involved. If allowed to exist, it can be destructive to any family.

Action

This is the time for you to be proactive and show your problem solving strengths. You can turn this situation around. Begin by exploring within yourself your concerns about fatherhood. Determine which concerns are keeping you from being part of your child's life.

The next step is to discuss your insights with your wife. Use her comments to help resolve your concerns. It is very likely that she will have some reasons that allowed this situation to exist. Understand those reasons and work to put them in perspective. Recognize that your goal is to have a rewarding relationship with your child as well as your wife.

Remember, you need your child's contact and your child needs the interaction and the nurturing that fathers are uniquely able to provide.

On a positive note, the simple fact that you are reading this book illustrates your interest to be involved in this pregnancy. It also supports your desire to become a great father right from the beginning.

Chapter Nine

. . . Action

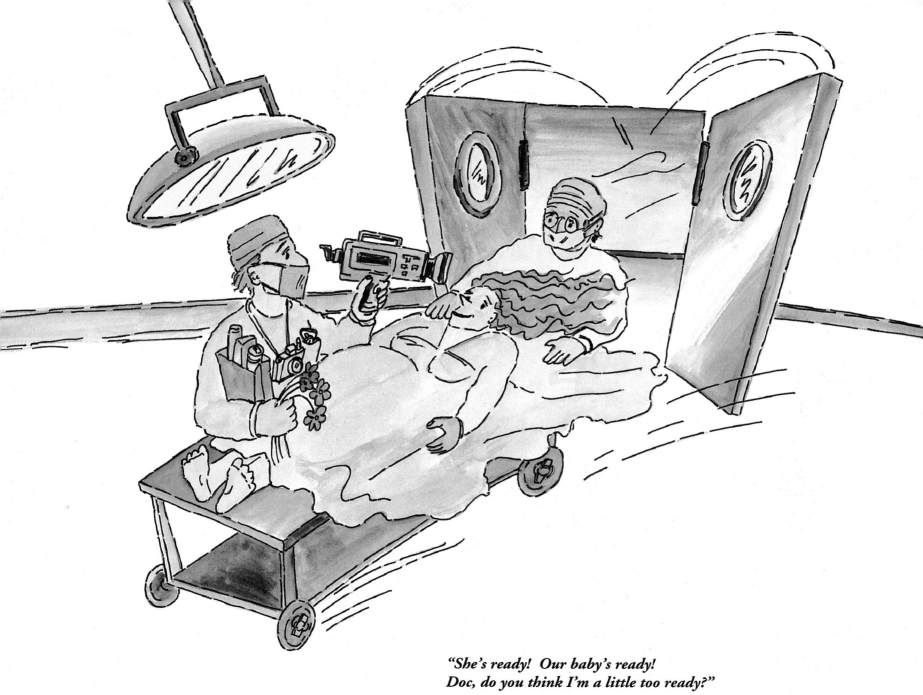

"She's ready! Our baby's ready!
Doc, do you think I'm a little too ready?"

This is it, Dad—the bottom of the ninth, fifth set and fourth quarter all rolled into one. This is the reason you've been getting ready—within yourself, with each other, at home, at work, with friends and family—for nine months.

This is childbirth.

The Beginning of Childbirth

A common question new parents have is, "How will we know when *it's* really beginning?" After all, there's a good chance your wife will experience contractions starting several weeks before her due date. That's normal, but that's not labor. It's your wife's uterus, which plays a major role in the drama ahead, loosening up for the real thing. There's also no predictable time lapse between false labor and the real start of childbirth.

It's probably the real thing when your wife's contractions become more frequent and intense. She may feel pain in areas beyond her back and her contractions may intensify when she walks around or repositions her body.

"But what if her water breaks?" you say. (That's when the amniotic fluid that surrounds the baby "breaks away" in preparation for childbirth.) "Isn't that a surefire sign?"

Pretty much, but only about one in six women experience this before labor starts. But don't despair. It's actually fairly hard to mistake the real thing once it begins.

That doesn't stop some men from being haunted by this possibility. They tell their wives where they are every minute. They strap themselves to a beeper or equip their wives and seventy-five close friends with cellular phones. I was typical, maybe even a little overboard. I put a phone in my car, had my secretary on alert, and started calling both home and office every few hours, wherever I was. I also cancelled *all* my travel plans.

You don't have to call a halt to your life a month before the due date. In fact, staying as close as possible to your normal routine can relax you and your wife. But it does make sense to have a few things well in hand several weeks before the "gun lap."

Checklist for Labor

This list assumes you've chosen a hospital birth to be supervised by an obstetrician— the most frequent choice of new parents. Here are some action items to accomplish:

• Help your wife pack her bag; don't forget things like extra socks in case your wife gets cold feet during labor, a washcloth, some books or magazines to while away the hours during early labor (my wife, always partial to fashion magazines, found these particularly helpful). And you might want to pack your own bag or add a few items to your wife's: magazines, snacks, reading from work (maybe a bottle of champagne and glasses?)—and, of course, a gift for your wife.

• Fill out as many of the hospital admission papers as you can before you actually need them, and keep those papers in a place where you won't forget where they are. When it's time to head for the hospital, the last thing you'll want to do is search for your papers, or (even worse) stand at an admitting desk filling them out. You might want to see if you can leave the completed papers at the admitting desk of your hospital or birth center so they're already on file when you arrive; if so, be sure to keep another set at home and take them with you. (In the worst case, you'd be filling out your papers with one hand while driving with the other.)

• Put your doctor's number right over your phone. He or she is the first person you'll want to call when you think your wife's contractions are the real thing.

• If it's not at an unreasonable hour, let a close friend know when you head for the hospital. Ask that friend to inform a few other key people.

• Keep your gas tank full. If you don't, labor is sure to arrive in the dead of night, and you'll spend precious minutes looking for a gas station as your warning light flashes.

• Have an extra set of car keys where you can find them in an instant. It's easy to misplace your keys just before you really need them.

• Make sure you know the shortest route to the hospital or birth center. Have an alternate route planned in case your main roads are clogged with traffic.

• You might want to make arrangements with a backup driver in case the unthinkable happens: your wife goes into labor and you can't get home to take her to the hospital.

• Have your car seat in the car. You'll need this in order to leave the hospital with your newborn.

When Do You Call the Hospital?

Most men learn about the start of labor when their wives say to them, in an unmistakable voice, "Uh, honey . . . I think it's time." In the stereotyped version, this sends the man into a well-meaning panic that renders him worthless (though he usually snaps out of it in time to be helpful). Usually his wife is a pillar of strength, as well as calm and efficient.

When your wife lets you know she's having contractions that seem like the real thing, it's time for you to stay calm and focused—which will help her do the same. If your wife is making specific requests or giving directions, it makes sense to follow them; if she's not, this is a great time for you to take the lead.

Your first job is to time the contractions, since the doctor will want to know how far apart they are. Contractions are timed from the start of one to the beginning of the next. Have your watch or stopwatch handy.

For first-time mothers, most practitioners will want you to come in when your wife's contractions are eight to ten minutes apart. It's probably a good idea for you, your wife, and your doctor to decide this beforehand. That way, when contractions begin you can start timing them right away.

If you have any doubt about what to do, you can always call your doctor or just go to the hospital. Maternity wards and birth centers see plenty of men arrive earlier than they have to, so don't worry about being embarrassed or looking dumb. What's the worst that can happen? They'll send you home with some calming, supportive suggestions.

How Labor Happens

There are four stages of labor. Although there can be tremendous variation, labor for first-time mothers averages about fourteen hours.

The *first stage* begins with the onset of contractions and ends when your wife's cervix is dilated to ten centimeters (about four inches). Getting her cervix fully dilated is what these contractions are for; your child arrives via the cervix. This stage has three parts we'll look at shortly.

The *second stage* begins when your wife is completely dilated and starts pushing your child through the birth canal; it ends when your baby is born.

I know, I know . . . your child is out and there are still two stages to go?

In the *third stage* your wife expels the placenta, the life-support organ that's vital to your child's survival in the womb.

And the *fourth stage* is recovery from the whole unforgettable and wonderful experience—physical recovery for your wife (maybe you, too!) and definitely emotional adjustments for both of you.

Once they're settled into fatherhood, many men recall the intensity of those first few hours. I remember being incredibly happy, tired, hungry (after fifteen hours without eating—be sure to pack some snacks in your hospital bag), and relieved all at once. I also felt a little scared by the delivery as well as by what laid ahead. But I was amazingly proud of my wife, in love with my daughter, and happy about what I'd contributed for the last nine months.

Before you get to feel that, Dad, there's labor and delivery.

A Look at Stage One

The first stage of labor has three parts: latent, active, and transition. Each is defined by the amount of dilation (in centimeters) that your wife's cervix has reached.

1) The latent or early stage starts with mild contractions that aren't necessarily happening at regular intervals and don't last more than about half a minute. During this phase your wife will be able to continue with her normal activities (unless she's in the middle of a triathlon). You can start to time her contractions and stay calm. Latent labor ends when your wife is dilated to three centimeters (or 1.2 inches). Now she's headed into active labor, when the contractions intensify and come more rapidly.

2) By now, if you're not at the hospital . . . *what are you waiting for?!* Active labor is also when your wife's water is likely to break, if it hasn't already. What new father can forget when his wife's water broke? For me that moment came at about 3:00 A.M., when I was awakened from a not-so-deep sleep to hear my wife heading for the bathroom to the accompaniment of gently but steadily dripping water.

"Guess what, honey?" she said in a perfectly calm voice. Then, I knew it was time. During active labor you're striving to be a "rock" as your wife's discomfort becomes more acute. With contractions intensifying and coming more regularly, she'll need plenty of encouragement and reassurance, delivered in a calm, steady voice.

But it's probably not a great idea to sweet-talk your wife while she's in the grip of a tough contraction. I learned this when my wife snapped at me in the labor room. You shouldn't take what your wife says during active labor personally. Expressing strong and even negative emotions or ideas helps her cope with the pain.

When dilation reaches seven centimeters (a shade under three inches), the last part of the first stage—transition—begins.

3) Transition is when most of the things that parents-to-be associate with labor happen. This is the "land of big pain" for your wife, when she's likely to express doubts about her ability to get through (and her comments might get even sharper). Her cervix is getting stretched to the ten centimeter mark, and the strain is likely to show over her face and entire body. It's at this point that I felt most useless. All you can do is "be there" as a calm and supportive partner.

Transition is difficult for your wife and likely to be the same for you. Many men are unnerved by what they see their wives go through and what they hear. You and your wife are likely to get annoyed if the medical staff isn't immediately responsive to your every request. I did; my wife was having major discomfort, to which they seemed indifferent. My wife was in terrific physical shape, thanks to plenty of running, skiing and some tennis, but she was in a great deal of pain. The arrangements we thought we had made for pain relief turned out to be news to the medical staff, who claimed that since it was Sunday they were having trouble locating an anesthesiologist.

My wife is rarely at a loss for words, and transition was no exception. She spewed major league venom. I was occasionally a target for some of this abuse and felt hard-pressed to keep from snapping back.

But while I remember how sharp her comments were, and how upset I felt, I couldn't tell you anything specific she said. My wife can barely remember talking that way about anyone during labor. That's the way it works. Memory protects us all, and it's worthwhile to keep in mind that people in extreme circumstances do and say things they'll readily disown later on. A woman in transition is definitely in extreme circumstances.

So no matter how tough it gets to watch your wife endure the pain . . . no matter how stinging (and seemingly sincere) her barbs may get . . . and no matter how irritated you feel over the incompetence of the medical staff . . . you need to stay focused on the goal, which is to help your wife with the delivery. That means encouraging and reassuring her, mopping her brow or rubbing her back, whatever it takes to get her through.

It's vital for you to stay positive and tell her how well she's doing, no matter how much unjustified abuse you're absorbing. If you have concerns you want to discuss with the doctor or nurse, do it out of sight and hearing range of your wife. When your wife reaches ten centimeters, transition is over and the second stage of labor is under way.

Stage Two: The Big Push

Just when you thought labor couldn't get any more difficult, it does.

The second stage is made up of pushing at the beginning and middle, and a new baby at the end. Your wife will start to feel pressure and an urge to push, which is "just what the doctor" (actually, nature) ordered. This is where you can use what you learned and practiced in childbirth class, as she gets into the rhythm of breathing, pushing, and relaxing. Remember to coach your wife to keep her hands open and flat. This helps force her energy to the cervix, where it's most needed.

Be sure you breathe as well. I got so involved in breathing with my wife, and was pushing along with her so hard, that I briefly passed out. That wasn't what her doctor had in mind for my role, but at least he couldn't doubt my involvement!

Your wife needs you to help her down the home stretch. She's likely to be very tired, but her contractions, although still powerful, may not be quite as painful. She needs to summon every bit of energy she has, and she'll need to draw strength and courage from you and the medical team.

Even what my wife had gone through in the first stage didn't prepare me for what came next. Every muscle of her body strained at the task. Her face contorted and her grunts were loud. She seemed unable to relax sufficiently between pushes. It was frightening, but a small consolation was that another woman two doors down was expressing herself much louder than my wife.

We got through it. Your wife also knows the end of her ordeal is in sight, and she may feel a surge of energy and resolve just before delivery. This is no time for you to let up. As birth gets closer, the medical team works closely with your wife, but you still play a big role. Encouragement and support mean more to your wife at this point than the clinical instructions she's getting from the medical staff. So keep telling her how well she's doing. As your baby starts to make his or her appearance, let her know she's "almost there."

And then, after what seems like an endless sequence of pushing, breathing, and groaning, it happens. Your baby says farewell to the only home it's ever known to meet Mom and Dad for the first time.

I've heard several new fathers talk about the awe they felt at seeing their wives in the grip of childbirth. For me, the awe was real but delayed. While my wife was going through labor, I was nervous and frightened, but working hard not to show it. I found out later that my wife greatly appreciated my apparent ability to stay calm and focused on supporting her throughout. To me it seemed like I hadn't done much beyond hold her hand, and rub her back and shoulders. I tried to reassure her as best I could, and keep my occasional questions to the doctor appearing casual. But when I heard how much she appreciated my support I knew I'd done a good job.

Congratulations, Dad! It's a safe bet you'll never forget the birth of your child. It's the most powerful blend of joy, relief, pride, and excitement you'll ever feel. I remember feeling a touch of pride in knowing that I'd made a difference and that all three of us had gotten through it together. We had a baby!

Still Two Stages to Go

Your baby is born, but labor isn't over. One of the first things the medical staff will do with your baby is give it a test—The APGAR test. It only takes a few minutes to observe and measure your baby's heart rate, breathing, skin tone, movements, and reflexes. Meanwhile, you'll be busy comforting your wife and sharing feelings that will overwhelm both of you.

Your wife's uterus is relaxing, too. But it has one more job to do—expel the placenta. This is the third stage of labor.

After what she'd been through, my wife barely noticed it when the placenta left the womb. I've heard other women say there was some pain and *more contractions!* Your wife might even have to resume some of the breathing techniques you thought you'd put behind you.

The medical staff wants to make sure all of the placenta makes it out, since leaving any behind can cause infection and bleeding. There's a good chance you (and even your wife) won't notice when this happens, since you'll be transfixed by your baby.

The fourth and final stage is recovery, which begins the minute your wife has lost the placenta. Now you have a chance to spend some priceless time with your baby. Your baby is likely to be quite active during the first hour or so after birthing, but will soon become very tired.

What happens to your baby is comparable to what you experience after a really long airplane flight. The thrill of arriving in a faraway place may give you an energy surge, but jet lag soon catches up. Entering the world is rougher on your child than even the longest airplane trip, so it's no wonder that he or she falls asleep soon after completing the journey from the womb.

On to Fatherhood

Labor and delivery are the climax—but not the end—of your thirteen-month journey. We haven't dealt here with cesarean delivery or any of the complications that can occur during childbirth. It's not that I want to minimize their reality; I feel your practitioner and childbirth class are the best sources of information on these topics, since those are the most personal and supportive ways for you to get the facts.

For now we'll assume that, as happens in the vast majority of cases, mother and child are doing well (you too, Dad). You and your wife are exhausted, but exhilarated. For nine months (maybe more) most of your attention and energy have been focused on childbirth. Maybe you haven't given much thought to what awaits you in the next four months. Our next chapter gives you some pointers for those first months as new parents.

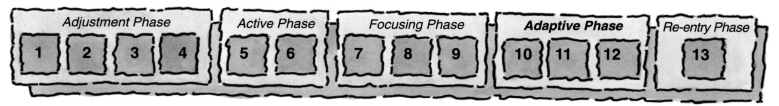

The "Adaptive" Phase

If you thought pregnancy was a big adjustment, wait until you see fatherhood!

Long after specific events fade from memory, most parents remember what these first months with their baby felt like. They were tired most of the time. Sometimes frustrated because of the baby's crying. They worried that maybe they weren't cut out to be great parents after all.

These reactions are very common, and it's a mistake to think that you and your wife will be able to avoid them completely. But a proactive approach to pregnancy can give you and your wife plenty of coping skills and a solid foundation for teamwork. This section looks at practical steps you can take to ease the impact of these first three months (chapters X-XII). And look on the bright side: You can't really understand how joyful being a parent can be until you experience it yourself. That's what awaits you in the next three months.

Chapter Ten

Common Reactions

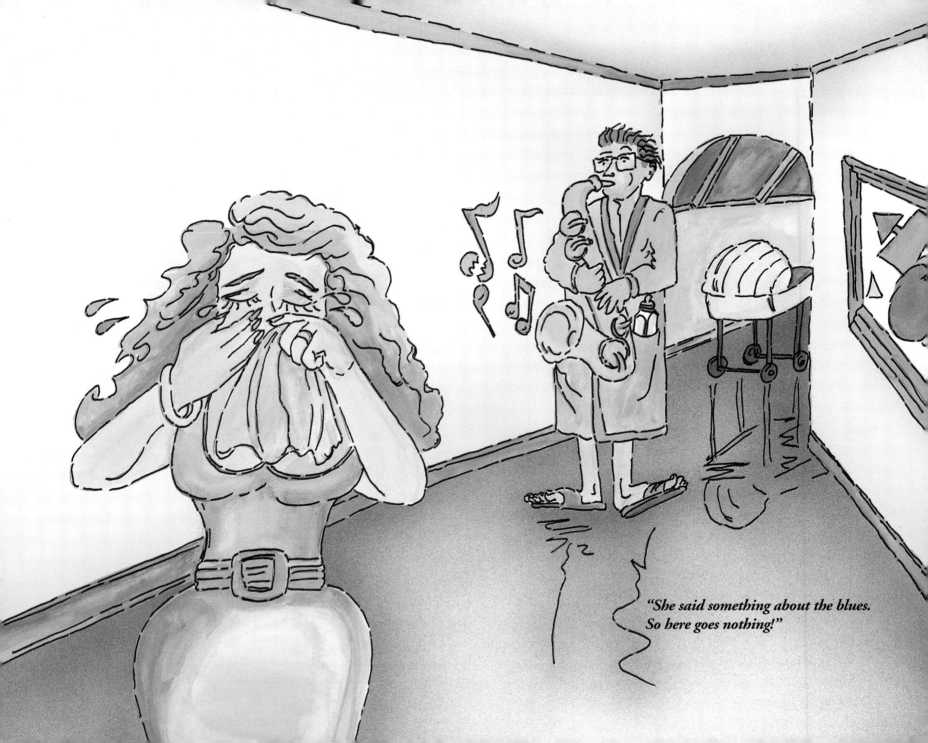

"She said something about the blues.
So here goes nothing!"

Believe me when I tell you, you are still pregnant! Only now you are giving birth to a new set of emotions and reactions you'll experience over the next four months. But it's the most enjoyable tired you've ever known. Many men are amazed by how quickly they become attached to their babies. You also feel phenomenally proud, protective, and tired. Even if your baby was to settle immediately into a routine of sleeping through the night (which probably won't happen), you and your wife would still have some adjustments to make. Now that parenting is a reality, your focus shifts dramatically to these changes in your daily living and during these first few months. It's okay to live one day at a time, because each day brings so many new, exciting, and unpredictable changes.

Adapting to these changes doesn't happen overnight. It takes time for all three of you to adjust to your new activities, routines and roles. When you do, you reach a new equilibrium in your household that feels different than, and at least as comfortable as, what you knew before. Four months is a reasonable amount of time to allow for this transition.

One of the best descriptions of parenting I've heard is that it's like taking a two-part course to learn to fly an airplane. During the first part, the instructor gives you the classroom theory with all of the books, charts, and lectures. He is also readily available to answer your questions. But for the second part, which includes the hands-on and actual flying, he simply hands you the keys, points you to the plane, and says, "Good luck."

This chapter covers some common reactions to being a new father, and how you can rise to the occasion. My goal is to help unlock your talents as a father and your resourcefulness as a husband.

Opening Night

I'll never forget our first night home as a family. Basically, our daughter cried nonstop. Every possibility of what could go wrong entered our minds. The more we tried to calm her, the more she cried.

Needless to say, we were at our wits' end, and at the doctor's office, at sunrise, even though it was a Sunday. The problem? Nothing that the doctor could find. The baby had just been crying all night.

"She's fine," the doctor said. I was shocked. That was the only possibility that hadn't occurred to us.

We were typically nervous new parents, and you probably will be, too. No amount of reading, talking, or classes can really prepare you for those first days. I was convinced I'd be totally inept. I'd already broken my own record for consecutive time spent with an infant. It was clear that our child had no concept of the importance of a good night's sleep for his father's career and mental health.

Later on I found out that these reactions are common—I wish I'd known! The "secret" is that, like most new jobs, the only way to learn it is to do it.

So don't worry! You'll be amazed at not just how quickly your child changes, but how quickly you'll grow into your new role. Much sooner than you'd imagine, you'll be handling those baby routines, quickly and efficiently, as though you've been doing them your whole life. This even happens to men who, like me, weren't sure they were really looking forward to becoming skilled at diapers. It just didn't fit with my image of myself somehow. My self-image changed quickly as I added the skills of a confident and competent father.

But that doesn't mean you'll bypass every possible pitfall. You might feel jealous or excluded as your child and wife bond strongly and your wife seems to have no time or energy for you. You may feel vaguely disappointed if labor and delivery didn't go as smoothly as you had expected. Whatever you experienced, the positive and lasting delights of your newborn will overshadow these temporary feelings or concerns.

It helped me to know and remember that my wife and child were learning as they went along as well.

Your Wife Bounces Back

During the first week at home your wife should rest as much as possible. Labor and delivery inevitably are a tremendous energy drain—the more she expended giving birth, the longer it usually takes her to recover. This recovery takes at least six weeks if she gets the rest she needs and doesn't waste her energy on unnecessary tasks. Otherwise it could take several months.

Healing for new mothers is emotional as well as physical. When your wife doesn't get enough rest, there's a good chance she'll be emotionally out of sorts and irritable. Being tired constantly also increases the odds that she will suffer mild depression. Lack of rest is a major contributor to these well-known postpartum blues, a fairly common occurrence among new mothers. (Only about 10 percent of new mothers experience genuine postpartum depression, a more severe condition.) So whatever you can do to minimize the emotional and physical demands on your wife will help speed her recovery.

That's why I recommend that you take some time off from work. This is a crucial time for you to carry more than your weight around the house. You won't be much good at work and you are needed much more at home.

Oddly enough, I went through a down period around this time as well. The meaning of "your life will never be the same" was starting to sink in. I hadn't been this tired since finals week in school. I felt frustrated by not knowing what the baby was crying about. But I took what I thought was the only reasonable approach—maintaining that positive attitude. My baby wasn't going away—thank

God—so I told myself to make the most of it, have fun, and look at it as a challenge. I'd been successful in my work and other endeavors that were important to me. My baby was the most meaningful long-term challenge I'd ever faced, and I was determined to be successful as a father.

Can We Make Love Now?

In the "good old days" most doctors were firm—no intercourse for six weeks. These days there's more varied opinion, but three weeks minimum is a good rule. That assumes, of course, that your wife is ready as well. Some women don't regain the sexual spark for weeks or months.

Don't take it personally, Dad, really. Who feels sexy when he or she is constantly tired, still recovering (maybe with stitches), and can't remember being anything but tired?

Making love might sound good to your wife if she has any energy left after all the other work is done. So make sure she doesn't have two people to mother! The faster you and your wife adjust to new routines and demands, the sooner you'll return to your normal love life.

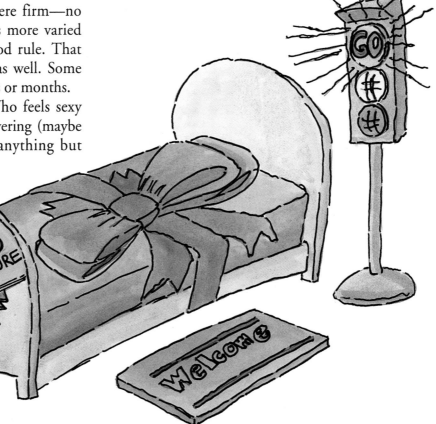

Here are some suggestions to make these first weeks as a parent easier:

• Simplify your household routine. You'll be amazed at how easy a baby makes it to loosen up in keeping your home white-glove spotless. Okay, so you can't let your house degenerate to the squalor of your first bachelor apartment, but don't be afraid to cut yourselves some slack. You might want to recruit your mother, mother-in-law, sister or (a close) friend to help you regain some semblance of order.

• Take over the kitchen and laundry room; if you're really ambitious, you could become your family's prime shopper as well. That's not a misprint, Dad! Remember that adjustments to "traditional" roles in the first few weeks aren't necessarily permanent. What counts now is getting the job(s) done. There's no such thing as "it's not my job" for you in these early weeks. This is the nineties, Dad!

• Control the flow of visitors. Friends, parents, and in-laws are of course dying to see the baby, but your first priority is your baby, wife, and self. A gentle but firm suggestion that another time might be better for a visit is not being rude.

• Pay close attention to your wife's moods and feelings. You can be her best defense against the blues. Don't neglect your own feelings, either. In fact, given the hormonal adjustments your wife is still making, your emotions are probably more manageable than hers at this stage.

• Set aside time for you and your wife . . . alone! And set some more time aside for you and your child . . . alone! One of the best ideas my wife and I ever had was designating a regular time when my wife was free to do whatever she wanted, and it was just me and my daughter, one-on-one. Now I wouldn't give that time up for anything. What can you do with your baby? Plenty. Why not visit with your parents or other relatives? How about seeing a friend from your childbirth class? Or you could take your baby for a "walk" to a nearby park.

• Find a new parent support group if you and your wife need to see other people who haven't slept in a month. Or call some of the people you met in your childbirth class to share war stories. Hearing other new parents describe the same traumas you're going through can really be reassuring. It also helps remind you that, no matter how tired or overwhelmed you're feeling, keeping your sense of humor is still vital to your sanity.

Chapter Eleven

Living in Harmony

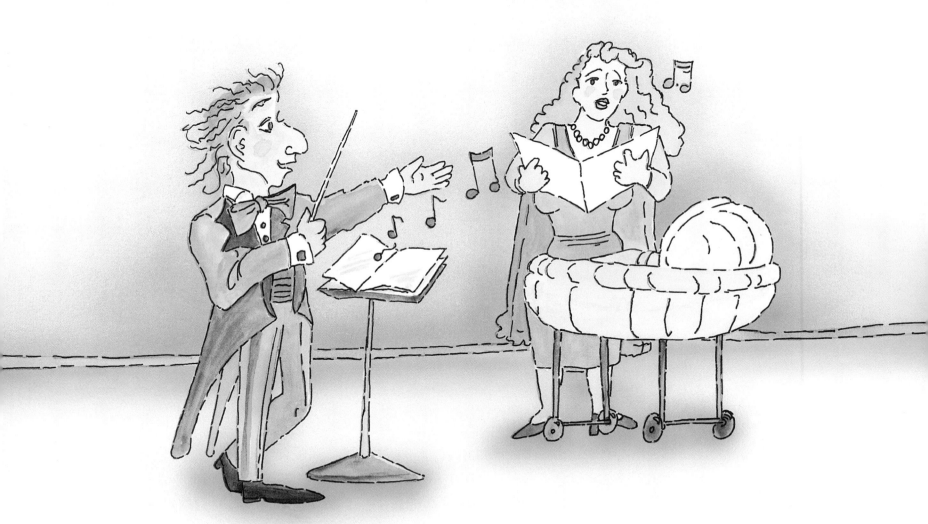

"A one-a and-a two-a and-a . . ."

I learned early—really early—that the keys to the last three months of the journey to fatherhood are patience, time management, and the critical selection of a pediatrician.

It was a gorgeous late-July day when I rode to the hospital to pick up my wife and three-day-old baby. I pulled up to the main entrance and waited for them to come to the door. "They'll be right down," I told myself confidently.

So I waited. And waited. I was getting irritated and edgy. Was there a problem? My eyes scanned the parking lot, anticipating a firm but polite reminder from hospital security that I couldn't just stand where I was.

More time passed. Now I was worried and angry. Where were they?

After thirty minutes I threw in the towel. I parked and walked up to the room. "Are you ready, honey?," I asked, trying to conceal my irritation. "I thought you'd be downstairs by now."

"Oh, I was just waiting for you," my wife said. "They won't let me come downstairs by myself. What took you so long?"

My anger disappeared with one look at my daughter. We drove home a happy family. The memory of sitting there stewing at the hospital parking lot faded quickly. That's too bad, because this little incident concealed lessons I was too preoccupied to learn.

First is the need for patience—with your wife, your baby, and yourself. (I'm not saying I should have waited any longer in the car, though.) The second is the danger of making assumptions about what your wife expects, needs, or feels. And the third is the need to learn that when you're a father, practically everything you do will take much longer than you figure—or than it used to!

Let's look a little more closely at these fundamentals for the first few months.

Patience Is a Virtue

Eventually you'll learn how much the word "parent" really covers. Why not work on it from the beginning?

The three most important people to be patient with are yourself, your wife, and your baby. You might want to leave a little patience in reserve for your in-laws, but that could be a long-term project.

Patience with yourself in the first months of fatherhood is just good sense. After all, it'll be awhile before you'll be changing diapers and clothes and getting bottles ready as easily as you tie your tie.

I was like many other fathers in those hectic first weeks—learning on the job and not fast enough, it seemed to me. I recall feeling frustrated and asking myself if I could really handle being a parent. Especially when our daughter would cry no matter how much I held, rocked, or walked her around.

This part of becoming a father—getting comfortable with the routine tasks—is a little bit like being a child.

Whether it was climbing that huge tree in your neighbor's yard or grappling with tough equations in algebra, there were things that seemed harder than they turned out to be—once you tried them. The tasks you'll face now are similar.

It's important to stay patient with the mother of your child as well. She'll need six weeks—minimum—to get her strength back. My rule for the first few weeks was that I was happy (or at least ready) to pitch in on whatever needed doing when it came to our daughter. Now, ten years later, that rule is still in effect! You'll be amazed at what you learn to enjoy when you do it with your child in mind.

So help your wife get all the rest she can. I had a big advantage in this—my wife is an extraordinary sleeper. If sleeping was an Olympic event, this woman would win a gold medal.

When your wife isn't getting her rest, it's important to stay sensitive to her mood swings. I vividly recall a reminder my wife gave me in unmistakable terms about two weeks after we brought our baby daughter home. I had reached the end of my still-short rope after about twenty minutes of crying by our little bundle of joy. "Hey!" my wife snapped after I asked innocently what I should do. "I'm as tired as you are. And don't you forget it!"

Finally, your baby deserves lots of patience as well. Newborns can be a real shock to men who are used to dealing mostly with business people. Work on the adjustment, and keep in mind that your child picks up your attitude and feelings from your tone and body language long before he or she truly understands them. The need to be a good role model starts very early.

It took me a while to grasp the fact that our little girl was just a creature of instinct, with no insight into or control over what she was doing. This dawned on me when she urinated on my arm as I was showing a friend how I mastered the quick change art of diapers.

Time Management

One of the first things you learn about successful time management is to prioritize. Management experts advise you to determine what's really important, develop a short list of key priorities for the day, week, and month, and focus on them.

When you're a new father, this list has one item—your baby. Of course, you still have a separate list for work and for yourself; they just don't include any goals that are attainable in the short term.

I'm not saying that being a new father entitles you to toss your career, marriage, friends, and former life completely overboard. It's just that you shouldn't panic or be surprised if you find yourself letting some things slide at work or at home. That's okay—won't all that stuff at work still be there when you get back? (Yes, and more of it, too!)

I learned four rules that will help you manage your time and keep your sanity in these early weeks:

1) **Get your rest, too. I made a big mistake the first two weeks. I figured I'd stay up a couple of hours later every night to keep up with that office reading. Big mistake: I assumed, incorrectly, that I'd actually be able to sleep every night. Try to nap when your baby does, no matter what time it is.**

2) **Give yourself—and your wife—time away from your baby on a regular basis right from the beginning. This was a major factor in my wife's ability to recover from childbirth and my ability to fend for myself with our daughters. Time with your wife, away from your baby, is also vital for reaffirming your relationship as a couple.**

3) **Avoid rigid schedules at all costs! Your baby will make a mockery of them anyway. But it is good to establish** some routines for bathing and napping (if you can make them stick).

4) **Review your family's priorities and goals for the next three to four months. Making sure that you and your wife are "in concurrence" helps reestablish order in your lives as you adjust to the new routines, demands, and realities of parenting.**

Choosing a Pediatrician

Earlier I suggested an approach to selecting your doctor to deliver your baby. The same suggestion applies here to your selection of a pediatrician.

It turned out to be even more selective about our baby's doctor than I had been about my wife's. Once you've seen your child, and felt that incomparable surge of love, protectiveness, and concern for him or her, chances are that you'll be highly discriminating also.

Fortunately, pediatricians understand this well. Virtually every parent they see is eager to make certain that his or her child will get the best care possible, that nothing will ever be overlooked, misdiagnosed, or mistreated.

So it's important that your pediatrician be able to reassure you about his or her experience, thoroughness, patience, and accessibility. Once again word of mouth is a great way to come up with candidates, and the doctor who delivered your child probably can make several good recommendations of pediatricians.

You can also get references from parents. My wife and I spoke to several close couples in detail about their doctors and found that even this level of research uncovered significant differences among doctors in their styles and philosophies.

Ultimately your choice will be derived from the pediatrician whose values are consistent with yours as parents. You will look for an up-to-date doctor who is patient and reassuring to both you and your child. You'll also want a pediatrician who understands the concerns and unique qualities of "new" parents and who has a good sense of humor, and is available, especially after hours, when you'll need him or her the most.

What's Up, Doc?

We were an "average" couple when it came to seeing the pediatrician for the first time. We went in about five weeks after our child was born. This was the first face-to-face contact we'd had with him since that first night home, but it was about the four hundredth time we'd spoken with him.

Those five weeks had been filled with sleepless nights, crying, and a couple of unexplained (and harmless) rashes. There was a fair bit of sharpness between my wife and I, and a growing conviction that we were destined for the cover of *People* magazine under the headline, "Worst Parents in America."

But that appointment was a milestone. No matter what horror story we threw at the doctor, he was calm and reassuring. His tone and manner told us that he'd heard it all before—at least that's how it seemed to us.

In addition to learning your baby's current height and weight, the first appointment is the time to find out about the schedule for your child's immunizations over the next several years. It's also an excellent time to ask those questions. Our doctor was the soul of patience—he'd probably heard all those questions many times before.

Chapter Twelve

From Fantasy to Fatherhood

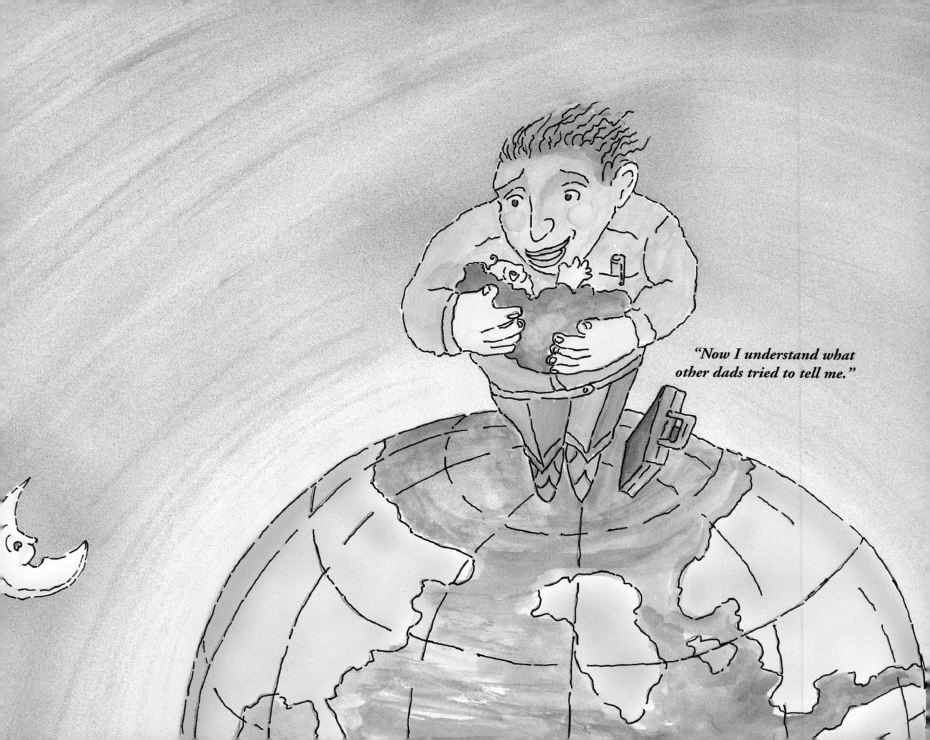

"Now I understand what
other dads tried to tell me."

Two or three months as a father will rid you of any illusions you may have had about parenting. Like most men, my fantasies skipped over the less glamorous parts— being a can't-miss target for spit up, for example. It left out lots of details about the great little surprises my child provided regularly.

But my fantasies also didn't include the best part— bonding with my baby. Bonding refers to the development of profound feelings of love, devotion, willingness to sacrifice, and protectiveness that a new father has for his child. Bonding also signifies the start of a relationship between you and your child. It is both physical and emotional.

Bonding is like hitting the ball on the "sweet spot" of your tennis racket. It's tough to describe but impossible to mistake for something else when it's happening. Many men assume that bonding resembles being struck by lightning— one dramatic event that changes you forever. They're wrong; bonding is a process by which powerful feelings develop gradually between you and your child.

During our pregnancy I had heard many men say, with complete sincerity, that being a father was the best thing that had ever happened to them. "Oh, it's changed my life completely," they would say, as a proud smile spread across their faces. "I'm really happy we did it."

I was looking forward to feeling the same way, and figured it would happen completely about three hours after our child was born.

It didn't, and in most cases it won't. My bond with my daughter took root when I cut the umbilical cord and held her right afterwards. That was a powerful *beginning* for my own bonding process, but that's all it was—a beginning. And that's the main thing about bonding—it takes time. There are occasional bumps in the road, but it will happen.

What kind of bumps? I remember feeling jealous of my child in these first months. After all, she seemed to be getting all my wife's love and attention, as well as that of our friends, parents, and complete strangers. To top it off, she was cutting deeply into my sleep.

Looking back, it's clear I had underestimated how long it would take my wife to bounce back and for us to develop a new balance in our lives. It's no surprise when you consider my ongoing fatigue and a heightened sense of pressure to succeed at work to make up for lost time. I also had some lingering apprehension about my ability to continue to pitch in on the routine tasks of parenting. It becomes clear why the now-rock-solid bond between my child and I didn't develop overnight, or as quickly as many men think.

But there were signs that bonding was indeed happening. The smile I'd break into whenever I looked at my daughter as she slept was the outward mark of the special feelings that were growing within me.

You'll have those same feelings. Time (lots of it) is on your side with bonding. As you and your family gradually settle into new routines, and as the rapid changes that your child goes through produce lots of delightful surprises, the bond will take root. Once it does, nothing on earth can shake it. That's because your child adds a new dimension to your life that makes you feel alive in ways you'd never have known about or imagined. Bonding is the process that brings those feelings into your life, forever.

Bonding Made Simple

A real milestone in bonding came for me when our first daughter was about ten days old. My wife had been a trooper through some long nights and tiring days, and she needed a break in the worst way. I couldn't say no, but I was worried: This would be the first time alone with my child.

Once Mom performed the mid-day feeding, she was gone. I was alone. No problem. I could handle anything, right? First couple hours she slept. I got plenty of work done around the house, feeling very productive and confident about my new role as Dad. Then she woke up and my first task was to change her diaper. I placed her in her freestanding windup swing in the middle of our living room as I tuned into the game. So far, so good.

Five minutes later, I heard a sloshing sound coming from beside me in the direction of my daughter. I turned toward her . . . I couldn't believe what I saw. The enclosed seat of the swing was filled with a runny brown liquid that would splash over the side with each move of the pendulum action swing. The carpet was a mess, my child (with an expressionless face) was up to her armpits in "diaper overflow."

I was motionless in disbelief. What should I do? What would Mom do? If I pulled her out, I would make more of a mess and risk dumping the contents of the seat on the carpet, and then what would I do with her? I didn't have quick access to a towel and I knew I had to act fast. I ran to the front door and threw it open. I grabbed the entire four-legged swing, being very careful not to spill anything. Lifting and moving quickly, yet cautiously, I managed to get the entire apparatus (with my kid still intact) onto the front lawn.

It was a hot afternoon, but even if it was cold out I probably would have done the same— I was on auto pilot. I grabbed the hose and made sure not to turn it on full blast. With one hand I unbuckled the safety strap that held her in place, submerging my hand in the warm dark liquid. It was the same hand that lifted her up and out of the seat. I held her over the lawn and hosed her down. I stripped her of her soiled garb and hosed her down again. Then, we went inside where I wrapped her in a warm towel.

I proceeded back to the front lawn were I squirted the swing until no sign of the event was evident. The carpet was next. Twenty minutes later, after using a variety of cleaning agents, the only evidence that was left was the dampness of the carpet. With the swing clean, dry, and in its place, I quickly placed the soiled clothes in the washing machine.

An hour later, everything was back in place. Her once filthy clothes, now clean and dry, were on her again. The house and child had no visible appearance of the disaster. Could I pull it off? Would Mom ever know that this happened? I watched the final minutes of the football game, thinking about how I handled the panic of the moment. I glanced over to my baby, once again swinging contently, and thought, if this is fatherhood, I can handle it.

Being a Father in the Larger World

A friend once told me a story that captures the adjustments you'll be making at work as a new father.

The atmosphere was electric. His manager had summoned my friend and two colleagues to an unscheduled meeting to clue them in on an organizational shake-up that had been rumored for weeks and was now happening.

His son was about six weeks old, and he'd put together an impressive string of near-sleepless nights leading up to the day of this meeting. He was tired, but not much more so than he'd been for weeks.

He sat down as far from his manager as he could. Not even her usual brisk tone could keep him from slowly nodding off into the sleep his body so desperately craved.

A co-worker tapped him lightly on the shoulder—he rallied. But it was a losing battle. The next thing he remembered was his colleague shaking him vigorously. Everybody was laughing good-naturedly. "How long was I out?" was the best line he could come up with. For those of us that are fathers we could easily relate.

Does anyone in that story sound familiar? The zombie-like appearance of the new parent at work is so common it's a cliche. After a while I learned that it's better to accept a certain level of fatigue than to fight it. I found that the best way to adjust was to tell myself in the morning, "Okay, you only slept three hours last night. Let's not push it today. Just focus on two or three things and get them done. Don't tire yourself out by moving faster than you have to."

Rather than fighting through the fatigue, I was able to accept it, almost work with it, and keep my goals realistic. I'd jump out of the shower feeling ready for the day—but not any less tired.

I tried to make the morning and early afternoon the most productive part of my workday. I'd devote the late afternoon to less taxing work—maybe catching up on phone calls or reading, and getting ready for my "second job" at home.

Even if you're getting your rest, it's very easy to feel distracted as well as tired during the first few months. You might find your thoughts wandering back (at any time *except* during the night) to the crib where your baby sleeps. You might feel an irresistible urge to dash home and play with your baby at the stroke of five—or you might not.

Whichever it is, that's okay! Trying to deny your feelings is as futile as trying to conquer fatigue by staying up later at night.

I found that a better strategy was to give in to the urge to race home at night and play with my baby.

A friend of mine gave me some great advice on this point about a week before I became a father. "Look," he said. "It makes more sense just to stick to an 8 to 5 work schedule for a few months, and let everyone at work know about it. That'll save you a lot of pointless worrying and phony excuse-making when you just want to get home to your child."

He was right. After all, if God wanted new fathers to put in late hours at work, would He have enabled people to invent voice mail, portable computers, or car phones?

Parenting, after all, is a change that ripples through everything—your work, your relationships, your life. The advantages of the take-charge attitude toward pregnancy that I advocate doesn't stop delivering benefits after your baby arrives. And taking charge means planning and teamwork.

Planning covers things like adjusting your schedules at work and at home, and trimming back your social life. Teamwork is the key to getting comfortable with the new routines, demands, and challenges that parenthood presents.

Let's look at how this works.

You're a Family Man Now

As I've said all along, an active approach to pregnancy offers rewards—confidence and readiness for the first months of fatherhood, for starters. The need for working closely with your wife doesn't end when your child arrives—it's just starting.

My own "rule," is that no task is too small—or "gender-inappropriate"—for a new father. My wife and I discovered some variations on this theme that served us well. At our home nobody did any one task all the time—(except for actual breast-feeding). Fathers should be generalists—comfortable doing any of the dozens of things that new parents need to do.

In those early months of fatherhood I fell into a habit that made cooperation easier. I'd stroll through the door, greet my wife and baby, and say, "So what's the plan for the evening?" I wasn't aware of it at first, but eventually I realized my question was an attempt to synchronize our plans for the evening. I was encouraging my wife to spell out those must-dos (dinner, feeding, some washing). We also discussed those want-to-dos (anything ranging from work-related reading to a nice long walk or an immediate dash for bed as soon as our daughter was asleep).

Eventually my wife started mocking me by saying "What's the plan?" just as I opened the door. But my tactic paid off; we usually had an agreed-upon approach to the evening. Of course, only about 4 percent of our evenings stuck to the plan. Okay, maybe 10 percent. But we were still ahead of where we would have been without it! And when I would come home with a plan for an evening out—with arrangements for a baby-sitter already made—my wife knew how much she meant to me.

The Joys of Fatherhood

Take a moment to reflect on the positive and exciting adventure fatherhood promises. It is a unique experience as you're already finding out. It's requiring all the skills of communication and the virtues of consistency and patience.

Think also about the importance that you play in your child's development. You've had an eager learner on your hands from the moment he or she was born. A child who is now growing emotionally and physically as a result of your paternal nurturing and through observing you as a role model.

This can be an exciting time if you take the time alone with your child to experience the joys of fatherhood.

Often we are so busy with our day to day lives and the tasks associated with a newborn that we forget to share what we enjoy in life with our children. Any time you take with your child to share your world will help build a foundation for a healthy father and child relationship. Be brave and consider the following for you and your baby alone:

- **Take baby on a picnic to the park or beach.**
- **Go to the zoo to watch the animals and the people.**
- **Strap on the baby pack and go for a hike.**
- **Take baby to work for a morning or afternoon.**
- **Do your around the house or garden chores with your baby with the pack on your chest or shoulders.**
- **Take baby to the aquarium, fish store, or pet shop.**

All of these opportunities give you a chance to enjoy your child in environments that you enjoy the most. Beyond sharing these experiences, you get the added benefit of showing off your baby and your skills as a father. Additionally, your wife will appreciate the break and take the much-needed time to herself to relax, regroup, or reflect.

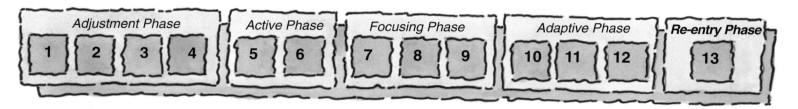

The "Re-Entry" Phase

The last phase of your thirteen-month journey arrives quietly. Maybe you'll get two consecutive nights of sleep for the first time since your child was born. You and your wife might decide to get a baby-sitter and go out on a date. Or you might stay late at work one night—just like in the old days.

These are signs that you've started re-entry. This begins around the time your child turns four months old, by which point your new roles and routines are well established.

You and your wife are a lot more comfortable as parents. The novelty of your status as parents is fading. Your friends and relatives recognize you are a family.

The thirteenth month is when balance starts to re-enter your life. Work, friends, and your own interests no longer take a back seat to the demands of parenting. Yes, Dad, there is life beyond parenting and the thirteenth month is when that life begins . . . again.

Chapter Thirteen

Back on Track

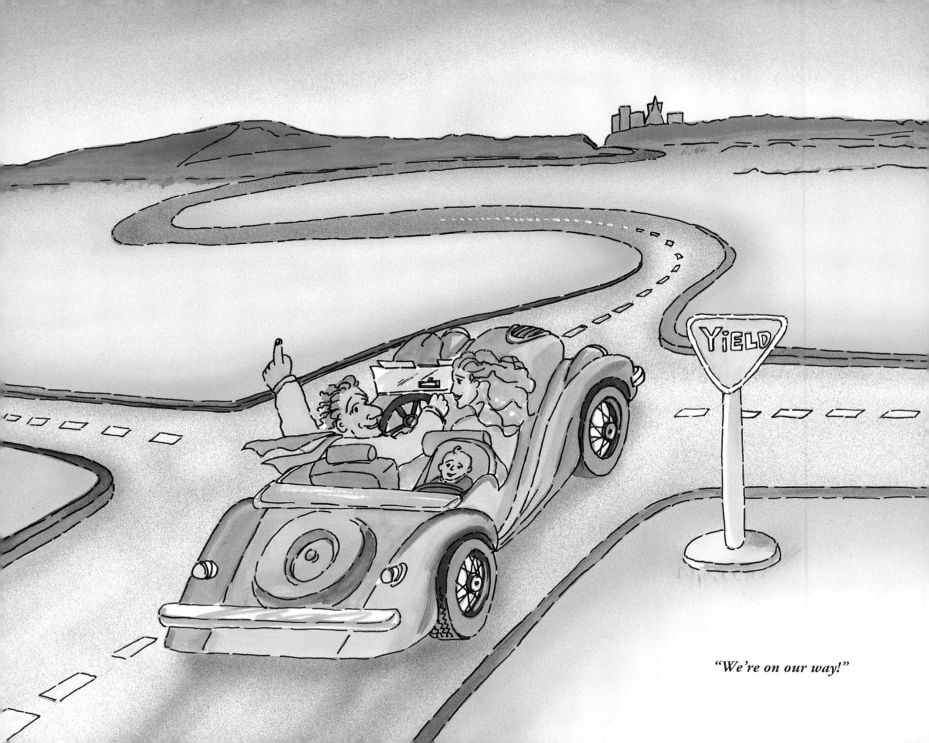

"We're on our way!"

Looking back at it now, more than ten years later, my wife and I called it "The Night from Hell"; it starred our daughter who wouldn't stop crying. At the time it seemed to be an intense event of global proportion. Yet in hindsight it proved to be small and singular experience of early parenthood. Thinking about that event awakened me to the fact that I made the adjustment to being a father.

Our girl was a little over three months old. She'd had a good day, and as always, we were hopeful that we'd somehow manage to get some "real sleep."

We'd barely made it from her room to ours when the crying began. We were a little surprised, since she hadn't shown any signs of getting sick or being uncomfortable.

We went through our usual routine of alternating who went into her room to check her out and comfort her. Soon it became clear that nothing was working or was going to. We were baffled. She didn't have a fever and didn't seem sluggish (in fact, she was crying with lots of energy). We thought about calling the doctor but decided against it.

The problem? Colic. It wouldn't be the last night of sleep we would lose to this condition, although our baby didn't suffer as badly as some children do.

The next morning (a workday) my wife and I tried to encourage each other over what passed for breakfast. I gave myself an extended version of my shower-stall pep talk; I was as ready as I was going to get.

It hit me when I was driving to work. For the first time, I didn't feel really put out or abused. I was focused entirely on my daughter, since at that point we didn't know what was wrong with her. My thoughts were not on how I would get through the day; they were on finding out what was happening at home and fixing it.

Looking back on that day about a week later, I realized that I'd reached a milestone. My life was getting *back on track*—it was the same track, really, but headed in a different direction. When my daughter got her first ear infection several weeks later, I was ready.

Virtually all new fathers reach a similar point around the four-month mark. You're getting more comfortable with the day-to-day tasks. You and your wife are settling into a routine and a division of labor. You're becoming less tired, since you can't remember what it's like to be rested. Business associates, relatives, and friends ask about your family before they ask about you. You're a father in the eyes of the world.

Around this time as well, if you've done all you could to help her rest, your wife's physical and emotional recovery is almost complete. You're getting caught up at work, thanks in no small part to your child's newfound ability to sleep through the night. There's probably even a spark of romance returning to your life, if it hasn't already. The return of your wife's sexual desire is the final indication that your wife has truly recovered.

In short, *balance* is making a comeback in your life. Your needs—personal, social, emotional, physical, and intellectual—are starting to reappear as priorities. You have whatever anxiety, doubt, and confusion you felt during pregnancy in perspective. Those were normal feelings, and any questions you had about either your ability or desire to be a great father have evaporated. *You're a family man.*

Reaching this point—and feeling good about it—is the payoff for taking an active approach since the day you learned you and your wife were pregnant. It's not the first such reward and it won't be the last; but it's important because it marks the end of a very tough adjustment to your new life. Your learning curve will never be as steep again.

Congratulations! Not only do you have all sorts of new parenting skills . . . baby stories to tell . . . and high hopes for the future, but you've most likely come to see your new identity as one of the best—and most significant—things about yourself.

Around this time I also noticed that something had changed between my wife and I. Deep down I'd known for a long time that our life together would never be the same, but I'd been slow to accept it. Now I knew we were going through something that was showing us things about each other we'd never suspected were there. We were a family, focused on a common goal. We were putting aside—temporarily, as it turns out—our personal pursuits (friends, sex, and exercise, to name a few) to work on that goal.

Being new parents had proven even more difficult than planning our wedding, an activity that had threatened our relationship at practically every turn. While there are still potholes in the road we're taking now, I realize that I couldn't dream of traveling it without my family. And for the first time, I'm not eager to move down the road at maximum speed. The journey truly is the reward; when you're not going as fast as you can, you see more along the way.

When I got to work that day, I knew I'd made the adjustment. I took an extra-long look at the pictures on my office wall. My motivation for doing well at work stared right back at me. Any resentment or pressure I had felt a couple of months ago was gone. Sure I still needed the recognition of my associates: that wouldn't change. But now I felt like I was a member of a different, smaller, more significant team. I was being dispatched to the work world as the family member best suited to put up with the steady flow of small annoyances without which work wouldn't be work. Now I reveled in the opportunity.

If you're lucky, if you take an active approach, and if you maintain a good attitude, you'll reach the same point as I. Most new fathers do. A family, it turns out, is far more than the legal relationships that define it; it's a stake in the future that no pension or portfolio can match. Now, when the phone won't stop ringing and those work emergencies pop up on every front imaginable, I sneak a glance at those pictures. It's the best way to keep work—and everything else—in perspective and in focus.

This new focus began when you recognized that you were creating much more than a baby when you and your wife were pregnant. You were also building a new identity as parents; pregnancy is the transition from your old identity to this new one.

If you approach pregnancy actively, you will end up with something very special—a deeper, more meaningful bond between you and your wife that is irreplaceable. And if you apply the idea that knowledge is power, you'll be ready to be the best parent you're capable of being from the first day of your child's life.

Congratulations! You've more than survived your thirteen-month journey to fatherhood. You've grown into a new identity that fits you well. Your proactive approach is paying dividends, and you're well prepared for the adventures that lie ahead. You'll never be the same . . . but you'll never want to be, now that you are experiencing *fatherhood.*

Relationship Update

This illustration depicts the ideal family whose interrelationships reflect balance. It symbolizes parents who are devoting the appropriate time and energy to their children, each other, and themselves. This illustration also suggests that both parents have a chance to develop common interests with their child. These interests come from the unique qualities each parent brings to his or her marriage and child. It is important that you and your wife give each other enough room to develop these interests.

What unites a family is the well-defined and clearly understood set of values and ideals the parents share. These core principles are a significant part of what parents give their children. These principles fuel their children's growth, allowing them to develop into confident, capable, and respected individuals. These values provide the strength and compassion to endure life's most difficult times as well as the joy and happiness to share the brighter moments. This type of relationship structure is the model for today's family.

Action

Make the development of this type of balanced family relationship your highest priority. Examine each of your individual strengths and build upon them as your most valuable assets to share with your child.

Recognize and accept that there will be some compromise in your couple's relationship, due to the addition of your child. Your ability and willingness to compromise (adjust your routine) can take you a long way toward meeting this ideal. You may not get exactly what you want initially, but the outcome will reward you and your family in new and fulfilling ways.

Glossary

This section of the book highlights the most common terminology used during pregnancy. I have avoided the use of such terms throughout this book, whenever possible, if simpler words were available. You may need to look up some of those words, often used by your doctor and most likely your wife as well.

APGAR score: Almost immediately after your son or daughter is born one of the assistants will determine your newborn's score. This score is a comparison to standards in five areas. They are: A-appearance, P-pulse, G-grimace (reflex), A-activity, and R-respiration. The test is performed again at five minutes to compare the previous observations. Each area receives 0-2 points, with a score closest to ten preferable. It is a little like counting toes, fingers, and limbs.

Braxton-Hicks contractions: This is the long name for "false labor." These are intermittent uterine contractions that may occur periodically during your wife's pregnancy. They cause the uterus to enlarge to accommodate your growing baby. Typically they are more frequent and sometimes painful as your wife approaches her "due date."

Breast: Larger than usual but only temporary. Sensitive, tender, and outright sore as baby adapts to his or her first bottle.

Cervix: The lower part of the uterus that will eventually dilate and thin out during labor to allow the passage of your baby.

Cesarean: This is a non-vaginal delivery that may or may not have been predicted in advance. For example, if a woman has a small pelvic opening and a large baby, or the baby is in a breech (feet-first) position, this would support a cesarean delivery. The doctor makes a surgical incision in your wife's abdomen and uterus to remove the baby.

Crowning: This refers to the appearance of the infant's head at the vaginal opening. About this time you're saying breathe, push, and anything else you can think of.

Dilation: This refers to the diameter of the cervical opening that ranges from 0-10 centimeters during labor. Ten centimeters is fully dilated and ready for delivery.

Effacement: This refers to the thinning, shortening, and drawing up of the cervix. At 100 percent the cervical canal has essentially disappeared.

Electronic Fetal Monitor (EFM): This is some of the "high-tech" equipment available to monitor and record the baby's heartbeat. It is also effective in measuring your wife's uterine contractions. Most men will become glued to the monitor that plots out a continuous curve and gives you warning of your wife's growing contractions.

Episiotomy: This is an incision in the area between the vagina and the rectum. It enlarges the vaginal opening and makes way for the baby. Not at all uncommon. After the baby is delivered the area is sutured and requires some additional healing time.

Placenta: Sometimes referred to as the "afterbirth" because your job and your wife's isn't over until this organ is eliminated after the baby is born. It requires some additional pushing. This flat organ in the pregnant uterus provides your baby's nourishment and eliminates its waste during the pregnancy.

Twins: Inspiration to work twice as hard all at once as opposed to spreading out the efforts and expense over time. But on the other hand they are twice the pleasure.

Uterus: Often referred to as the "womb." It is a pear-shaped organ that houses the baby, placenta, and amniotic fluid. It greatly increases in size and capacity during pregnancy and slowly shrinks to a smaller size in the weeks after birth.

References

Entries are listed in the order that they are mentioned in the text.

- **Family, Work, and Self,** Anne Pedersen and Peggy O'Mara, editors, John Muir Publications, 1990
- **From Here to Maternity: A Guide for Pregnant Couples,** Connie Marshall, R.N., Prima Publishing, 1991
- **When Men Are Pregnant**, Jerrold Lee Shapiro, Impact Publishers, 1987
- **Pregnancy: The Psychological Experience**, Libby Lee Colman and Arthur D. Colman, Farrar, Straus and Giroux, second edition 1991
- **Pregnancy and Birth Book,** Dr. Miriam Stoppard, Ballantine Books, 1985
- **What to Expect When You're Expecting**, Arlene Eisenberg, Heidi Eisenberg Murkoff, and Sandee Eisesnberg Hathaway, R.N., Workman Publishing, 1988
- **The Well Pregnancy Book,** Mike Samuels, M.D. and Nancy Samuels, Summit Books, 1986
- **Expectant Fathers,** Sam Bittman and Sue Rosenberg Zalk, Ballantine Books, 1978
- **Pregnant Fathers,** Jack Heinowitz, Prentice Hall Press, 1982
- **"The Expectant Father,"** Jerrold Lee Shapiro, *Psychology Today,* Jan. 1987, p. 36
- **"The 'Pregnant' Father,"** Robert McCall, *Parents Magazine,* July 1988, pp. 188-90
- **"Vomiting and Nausea in the First 12 Weeks of Pregnancy,"** George M. Iastrakis et al., *Psychotherapy and Psychosomatics,* Oct. 1988, Vol. 49, (11), pp. 22-24
- **The Father Book: Pregnancy and Beyond,** Rae Grad, et al., Acropolis Books Ltd., 1981
- **"Coitus and Associated Amniotic Fluid Infections,"** Richard L. Naeye, M.D., *The New England Journal of Medicine,* Nov. 29, 1979, pp. 1198-1200
- **"Becoming a Father: A Review of Nursing Literature on Expectant Fatherhood,"** Sister Corinne Lemmer, *Maternal-Child Nursing Journal,* Fall 1987, pp. 261-275
- **"Three Phases of Father Involvement in Pregnancy,"** Katheryn Antle May, *Nursing Research,* Vol. 31, No. 6, Nov.-Dec. 1982, pp. 337-351
- **Maternity and Gynecologic Care**, Margaret Duncan Jensen and Irene M. Bobak, The CV Mosby Company, 1985
- **Pregnancy and Parenting**, Phyllis Noeranger Stern, editor, Ohemisphere Publishing Corp., 1989
- **"Laboring for Relevance: Expectant and New Fatherhood,"** Pamela L. Jordan, *Nursing Research,* Vol.39, No. 1, Jan.-Feb. 1990, pp. 11-16
- **"Transition to Parenthood: How Infants Change Families,"** Ralph La Rossa and Maureen Mulligan La Rossa, Sage Library of Social Research, 1981
- **Fatherhood Today: Men's Changing Role in the Family,** Phyllis Bronstein and Carolyn Pape Cowan, editors, John Wiley and Sons, 1988